4/9/24 - hop

ELSBETH

In recording the dialogue and events in this book, much cross-referencing and concern for accuracy has been shown. Elsbeth approved all chapters, and David meticulously worked through manuscript, galley, and page-proof stages. Doctors and other participants reviewed the manuscript. The author apologizes for any inaccuracies which may remain.

ELSBETH

Harold Myra

FLEMING H. REVELL COMPANY
Old Tappan, New Jersey

Unless otherwise identified, Scripture quotations are from the King James Version of the Bible.

Scripture quotations from The Living Bible, Copyright © 1971 by Tyndale House Publishers, Wheaton, Illinois 60187. All rights reserved. Used by permission.

Scripture quotations from THE NEW INTERNATIONAL VERSION, Copyright © 1973 by New York Bible Society International, are used by permission.

Library of Congress Cataloging in Publication Data

Myra, Harold Lawrence, date
    Elsbeth.

    1. Cancer—Personal narratives. 2. Christensen, Elsbeth. I. Title.
RC262.M9   362.1'9'615500924   [B]   75-29472
ISBN 0-8007-0778-8

Copyright © 1976 by Fleming H. Revell Company
All Rights Reserved
Printed in the United States of America

Contents

1 Three Countries 9
2 Biafra 27
3 Two Weeks in the Bush 39
4 Together 71
5 Train to Serikin Pawa 83
6 An American Autumn 89
7 Lausanne 107
8 A Weekend in August 119
9 The Light 135
10 Afterward 155

ELSBETH

1

Three Countries

MOROCCO

"Mademoiselle! Mademoiselle!"

Elsbeth increased the pace of her walk as the number of French soldiers following her grew to nearly a dozen. As far as Elsbeth knew, she was the only European girl in Marrakech, Morocco—and the French troops were persistent.

How easy it would be to lose all my morals here, the Swiss girl thought as she briskly, determinedly kept ahead of her pursuers. Morocco was dangerous for a beautiful seventeen-year-old girl. It was now about ten in the morning. She had gone to the store to buy meat, but at night she would not go out in the streets at all. She hurried on to her great-aunt's tea shop, opened the door without a backward look, and entered, putting the Frenchmen out of sight and mind. Renee, the young Jewish woman in charge of the shop, was standing by the counter. Elsbeth liked working with her, learning the prices, and helping to sell when it got busy. In addition to the gift shop items displayed in the outer windows and on shelves, there were four tables with chairs for the customers who could buy cakes, pies, and pastries to go with their coffee or tea.

Elsbeth noticed Renee's black, wavy hair was bluish in the morning light. She was smartly dressed and had fair skin and dark brown eyes. They began laughing about the dolefulness of the French soldiers, then drifted to talking about Renee's family. In the mirror Elsbeth noticed her aunt walking toward the shop, looking far more like a soldier than the Frenchmen had, her head erect, shoulders back, full of purpose. Both girls grabbed dust rags and started taking down mirrors. "You should always be doing something," her aunt had insisted to them. "Never sit down. It's good for the customers to see you busy." The small, chunky woman with short-cropped, curly hair marched through the front door and began ordering them around. It was mid-December, and the busy Christmas season had begun. Antoine, the man her aunt lived with, had five Arab workers in the back of the shop making cakes, tarts, and pies.

Elsbeth looked at her stern aunt. The older woman had come to Berne a short time ago and invited her to visit here to master French. She was overweight, but had an attractive face and kept herself meticulously well-groomed. It irritated Elsbeth that her aunt felt herself so much more respectable than others. Everyone called her Madame Dépiez; but she had never married Antoine, though she'd lived with him nearly twenty-five years.

The next morning Elsbeth shivered as she got out of bed, even though a little gas oven was burning in her room. December in Morocco is cold, and there was no central heating in the one-story tea-shop home. She pushed the hide-a-bed back into couch form and did her daily ritual of precisely arranging her aunt's old-fashioned dolls on it. This room served as Elsbeth's bedroom, but then became the living room and dining room as well.

A *fatima*—an Arab servant woman—came in to set the table for breakfast. She bowed as she entered, and Elsbeth felt awkward. Whenever she could, Elsbeth sneaked the fatima some of the day-old cakes and pastries that her aunt would waste—rather than "spoil" a servant. Elsbeth and her aunt sat down at the table; everything around them was flawlessly arranged. They ate moon-shaped cakes and crescent rolls with tea. The fatima bowed and left obediently.

"I had a strange dream last night," Elsbeth told her aunt. "In the dream someone had died, and we closed the casket."

The older woman almost stood up from the table, interrupting her niece. "Dying! Elsbeth, why are you talking about dying? You are far too young to think about that."

Elsbeth was startled. "Why can't we talk about dying?" She was not afraid of her aunt. She stared into her large, blue eyes which glared down over a straight, strong nose.

Three Countries

"We are alive!" her aunt retorted. "We think of living, not of dying. After this life, it's finished. It's over. A young girl like you should be thinking of *life*."

"Well, I believe in life after death. Jesus Christ died so we could have eternal life. I believe in heaven."

Elsbeth's aunt gave her a withering look. The older woman—who read widely in four languages—considered her view the only intelligent one. "Huh!" she finally retorted. "You are too young to understand this. But you will grow up."

The fatima brought them more pastry as Elsbeth watched her aunt sip her tea. Madame Dépiez had left Switzerland at the age of sixteen for Egypt, had never married, but had had a child. She reminded Elsbeth of the stone of a peach, all tough and gouged—but with a good seed inside. The aunt returned her niece's affection, but Elsbeth wondered when she might smash against that rough exterior.

The teenage girl from Switzerland found she was developing a love for Morocco's people. The city of Marrakech was just sixty miles from the Atlas Mountains which separate the Sahara from North Africa. Its people were strictly separated, with Arabs living in one area, Jews in another, and Europeans in a third area. Elsbeth had visited a family in the Arab section. After work one day, she accepted Renee's invitation to visit her family in the Jewish quarter. They got into Renee's small car and drove past the two-story homes and beautiful yards of the European sector. Elsbeth noticed orange trees and, occasionally, Arabs riding on donkeys. But as they rode on, what struck her was the suddenness of the sunset. She looked up through the windshield and saw the stars and moon. The sky was black except for a streak of colors above the horizon; there was a dark-blue area, then violet, then bright orange, then yellow, then a rich, fire-red hue. Palm trees were silhouetted against the wide band of sunset colors.

The girls came to an older part of town and went through a gate. This was the Jewish section, and immediately, everything changed. The road was rough and potholed. Instead of homes, Elsbeth saw mud walls along the road. The walls had little entrances, and people would have to duck to enter. Men with beards and old, dark hats and women wrapped in bright-colored cloth bustled hurriedly past the traders sitting at tables and the children screaming to each other. The Jews had lighted their petrol lamps on the sales tables along the road, for there was no electricity in this part of Marrakech.

They parked and Renee unlatched her door. "Is the car safe here?" Elsbeth asked.

"Oh, yes," Renee answered as they got out. Elsbeth followed her through the little hole in the wall and was surprised to emerge in a lovely, open-air courtyard where there were wide-leafed, well-tended plants, and fruited lemon and orange trees. Rooms faced into the courtyard.

Renee's father was a prosperous trader and knew Arabic and a little French, with which he greeted Elsbeth. Her mother simply nodded pleasantly; her head was wrapped in a scarf as she prepared dinner over an open fire. They then sat on the floor on embroidered cushions near the fire and ate from a big plate. Elsbeth found the chicken and vegetable sauce with pepper and other spices uniquely delicious.

Elsbeth tried to make the most of her Morocco trip; she started attending a small church where she met a Swiss missionary who lived in the Arab sector. A French family from church invited her over to play the piano at their home. A rugged, British midwife ran a Sunday school and recruited Elsbeth to teach. She often spent an hour or two praying in a nearby church and felt very close to God. Yet she still had time to crochet, work in her aunt's yard with its lemon and orange trees and Granaud apples, and to play with the dog. A young French soldier from church drove her to a ski party in the Atlas Mountains.

But she became bored in Marrakech. At home in Berne, she was used to a regimen of hard work. Here she was even told not to do dishes. One Sunday, before church, the British midwife, tall, thin and sturdy, asked her in her rugged voice, "Look, Elsbeth, what are you actually doing here in Morocco?"

"I'm on a visit to learn French," Elsbeth replied.

"Can you do what you want?" The words were clipped in a distinct British accent.

"Why, they don't need me at all! I would love to be more useful."

Elsbeth was a bit in awe of this woman in her forties who seemed to accomplish the impossible every day. On a previous Sunday Elsbeth had asked how things were going and she had replied, "Well, I have six women in labor." During the church service someone had called her, and she had ridden off hurriedly on her bicycle.

"We have hundreds of Arab women coming with their children," she explained. "You could show them how to wash the babies and boil the water. You could help with the powdered milk. But especially we must emphasize they are to boil the water. Then we weigh the babies . . . ."

"Oh, of course I could do that!" Elsbeth was so thrilled she could hardly sit through the church service. She thought about the beautiful, light-bronze children with their black hair. As soon as the service was over, she half walked and half ran back to the shop.

She found her aunt in the store, working. Elsbeth rushed up to her, bubbling with excitement as she explained the need and the wonderful opportunity. "What do you think?" Elsbeth asked.

Her aunt was standing erect like a queen, and Elsbeth noticed her hands had tensed. "What do I think!" she exploded, as if she were about to grab a whip. She put her hands on her hips as Elsbeth wondered, *It's as if I'd reached over to rob her jewelry.* "Uh, huh," her aunt snorted. "You would like to go to those dirty, black kids. Could you imagine what people would think? Madame Dépiez's niece going to those dirty people? Absolutely no! Never!"

In the little room to the side, customers were seated at tables having hot drinks and rolls. They watched the exchange impassively, and though Elsbeth and her aunt were speaking Swiss German, the angry face and clenched hands carried the full force of emotions to the customers. But Elsbeth was less embarrassed than furious. She fought the desire to strike out and scratch her aunt's face. *How despicable,* she thought, *she who is so prim and proper and pretends she's married, when she's not.* Elsbeth could not believe the fire in her aunt nor the anger in herself. Outraged, she huffed to her room and then wept.

"Lord," she prayed, "I would love to help these people. I'm going to go home and learn my profession. I'm going to be independent from aunts and anybody else. Lord, let me help kids like that . . . ."

SWITZERLAND

It was several years later when Elsbeth was a student nurse that she met Claus. A doctor had invited several of the staff and students to his home on Lake Constance for a "musical evening." Claus, a young extern from Germany, had played the flute. During refreshments, Elsbeth walked down to the lake among small groups of people, and Claus deliberately aimed his feet in her direction. "I'm happy you were able to come," he greeted her.

"What's your name?" Elsbeth asked. She had seen the young doctor at the hospital.

"Claus Peter."

"Do you have any brothers or sisters?"

"Only nine brothers."

The wry understatement matched the merriment in his eyes. He spoke with a humble, but bemused, irony that immediately delighted Elsbeth. As they talked she learned that his father, a doctor, had been held by the Nazis in a concentration camp for six years while his mother had taken care of their boys. All during the war she had provided for them by doing underground translation work for the Americans.

The natural attraction between Elsbeth and Claus began building as they exchanged stories till past midnight. Finally Claus offered to walk her home. Elsbeth lived on the lake, which is part of the border between Germany and Switzerland. They walked around the lake until they arrived at her house. "Why don't we talk some more?" Claus asked as they stood in the moonlight. It was idyllic, a fairy-tale scene, complete with thick forests, hills covered with grapevines, and even an old castle in the distance. Elsbeth felt she was part of a romantic poem; there were swans on the lake and soft, bright moonlight touched the trees, the water, and their faces.

They decided to go back to a little island of trees where they sat on a simple bench made of a piece of wood and two poles. They held and kissed each other. They talked. The swans were motionless against the shore, the moonlight outlining their white shapes in the early summer night.

Elsbeth got a few hours sleep that Sunday morning before Erwin, a young man she had been dating for over a year, was to arrive. Shortly after her Morocco trip, she had made the mistake of not wanting to hurt a boy and had actually ended up engaged to that boy. However, they had broken up, and she had not become nearly as serious with Erwin. Now she knew why. She liked him a great deal, but she did not love him.

She was gentle, but clear, with Erwin. Yet her words, though phrased gently, came at him like little butcher knives. His dismay reached his face, and he began to break down in front of her, then started crying softly like a child. Elsbeth knew he loved her in the same way she now knew she loved Claus. Yet she couldn't return that love, even though she cared about him deeply. She couldn't possibly pretend.

The sharp sadness of the breakup scene mixed crazily that day with her desire to tell everyone about her magical evening. But in the rigid nurses'-training program, she couldn't let her supervisors know she was in love with a doctor she worked with. She told only Margaret, her best friend.

Claus and Elsbeth worked side by side, day after day, and no one suspected. One day she knew that Claus was on the second floor, practicing his flute in the bathroom so he wouldn't disturb anyone. Elsbeth was on the first floor in charge of two wards but furtively escaped, ran up the stairs, opened the door, kissed his shocked face, and ran down the stairs again, chancing that none of the other nurses or doctors would see.

Elsbeth and Claus swam in the lake. They read aloud to each other from *The Little Prince* by Saint-Exupery. One evening they went for a long walk. The hospital faced the lake; behind it was a hill, then a forest on the German side. They walked under a bright, full moon. In the middle of the forest they came to a little clearing, and there they sat, surrounded by big trees, feeling very romantic. The moon was bright enough to see the pages, so they began reading aloud the fox story from *The Little Prince*. It was past midnight now, almost as idyllic a night as the first night they'd met. Cricket chirps blended with the night sounds.

Suddenly they heard a loud panting, as if giant dogs were right behind them. *Huff. Huff. Huff.* They jerked around and edged back in disbelief. A huge, dirty, gray thing with long, menacing, white tusks and thick, ugly jowls was glaring at them, making fearful sounds. Behind the huge boar were a couple dozen gray shapes coming out of the forest and ready to run them down.

Claus grabbed Elsbeth's arm and they started running through the forest. The wild boars crashed and panted heavily behind them, following them around the trees and through the underbrush. They ran and ran and ran, finally breaking out to the edge of the forest. The boars were behind them somewhere, and they now walked more easily as they came into town. A field of wheat had just been cut and smelled fresh and inviting. They collapsed on the ground, then looked at each other, still shocked. This cannot be. Wild boars! The next day Elsbeth wanted to share her little adventure with everyone. But how could she explain her being out in the forest clearing—at midnight— to the prim matrons? Only Margaret got the details.

Claus returned to Germany, and Elsbeth was graduated. Later she traveled by train to spend Easter week with Claus and his family. They lived in a large home out in the countryside, where the father had a busy practice and the mother led a vigorous life of coordinating her family of twelve. Once a week they would have an evening concert in their home to which they'd invite patients and friends. Claus, his parents and brothers, all played in a gifted manner. It was just the sort of family Elsbeth pictured Bach as having had. Claus's father seemed a perfect caricature of a professor. He was short, bald, and wore old-fashioned glasses.

Elsbeth grew to love Germany with its gentle mountains. Unlike the Alps, she could see over them, far into the distance. She and Claus took long hikes and read to each other. On Easter Sunday they rose early and went to the little grave of Claus's sister. It was foggy. They stood at the gravesite wrapped in the fog for a while, then walked slowly to the church. No one had climbed its high tower for a very long time, but they persuaded the sexton to open it for them. As they got to the top and looked above the fog over all the newly green countryside, Elsbeth thought of Mary's coming early to the grave of Jesus. He was the Resurrection and the Life. Someday they would see Claus's baby sister who had died! Bells began ringing

Three Countries

from all directions from the many little villages surrounding them. Easter! Resurrection! Life!

That morning they attended the dedication service for the family's first grandchild. The week was becoming one of those fairy-tale dreams again, as Elsbeth fell in love with the family as well as Claus. But on Wednesday Claus had to take her on the eight-hour drive to the train station for her return to Switzerland. They arrived at the station early, so they went for a walk through a forest. It was foggy again. All they could see of the sun was a few beams penetrating the trees. The week had been almost too good, too wonderful. What would the future hold? "Well, I'll be coming to Switzerland soon," Claus said. "And in a year or so we'll be married."

Elsbeth finally boarded the train and settled herself on a seat by a window. As she watched Claus standing in the station, she felt lonely for him already. *But,* she thought, *we will see each other again soon. Soon.*

The first three days back at work were dull gray. The only color and verve was a letter from Claus. He wrote of how much the week together had meant to him and what she was becoming in his life. He quoted a poem from Goethe.

Four days after receiving the letter, a three-minute phone call from Claus devastated her life. She heard incredible words like, "I don't know how to tell you, but I want to stop our friendship. I can't explain it on the phone, but I just know we should stop." And then they were saying good-bye to each other, and she found herself with the mute phone in her hand, staring incredulously at it.

The terrible days following were filled with a snowstorm of questions. Claus wrote another letter, this time trying to explain himself, saying Elsbeth was way ahead of him spiritually. He wrote of their differences, yet said he still loved her. Elsbeth knew Claus had read all of Kierkegaard, that he had depressions and struggled, seeking answers which eluded him. She knew he prayed but didn't find peace. Could that be the only thing that had caused his turnabout? Wouldn't that make him want her more?

Elsbeth prayed and tried to accept it. This had been the first time she had loved a man—had fully trusted a man with her future, her thoughts, and her life. She did not feel bitterness. But the knife had sliced so deeply she was convinced she could never love again. From then on, she gently rebuffed any man who tried to win her attentions.

NIGERIA

The flight was scheduled to leave Zürich at midnight. Almost five years had passed since her breakup with Claus. She had since trained as a midwife and studied in England. Now she was heading for Nigeria as a medical missionary.

Elsbeth handed her winter coat to her mother, kissed both parents, and walked out to the plane. The snow whipped against her dress with the early April cold. Inside she sat down beside a Dutch woman who was flying to Johannesburg to visit her son. "Where are you going?" the older woman said.

"Kano, Nigeria," Elsbeth answered.

When the Dutch woman learned she was a missionary midwife who would be working out in the bush for two years, she protested several times, "Oh, I just can't believe that." Elsbeth did not have the stereotype, missionary-to-the-bush-station look. The two women literally talked all night, and it took Elsbeth's mind off the pain of departure. Being gone from home and from Switzerland for a full two years seemed like a huge, emotional mountain in front of her.

At six in the morning they landed in Kano, the first large city right below the Sahara. As soon as Elsbeth disembarked from the plane, she started perspiring. She saw black people everywhere. In Switzerland, if she saw one black man everyone would be turning around with her, looking. Here they were talking in Hausa and pidgin English, neither of which she understood. When Elsbeth reached customs, a Nigerian looked at her luggage. "Oh, a tape recorder," he observed. "That will be twenty-five pounds for the customs."

"Whaaaat!" Elsbeth demanded. She was tired, very hot, and anxious to get through, but she wasn't going to pay that much. She argued vigorously. Another customs official came and argued with her. After about twenty minutes, both men left to confront other passengers. "Lord," Elsbeth prayed, "You have to help me on this. I can't pay that much. Two or three pounds, okay."

"Look," she explained, "I'm going to a mission station in the

North. I'm just going to listen to the music—I'm not going to sell it."

"No," the man insisted in broken English. "Twenty-five pounds."

He let her stand there as he went off to deal with other people, then he came back. "Well, do you have the money?"

"No, I'm not going to pay."

After letting her stand there awhile, the man finally said, "Go." Relieved, she walked through.

A Swiss, Mr. Kunzli, picked her up. As they drove across Kano, its utter flatness and the smells of the sand and peanuts made her feel as if she'd landed in a different world. At home winter snow had covered leafless trees and barren ground. After passing through dry brushland, they arrived at the Kunzli compound. Elsbeth was amazed at how Kano's easily tapped water supplied green trees and grass and colorful flowers and shrubs on the compound. African flowers Elsbeth had kept in pots at home grew here in profusion.

They sat at an outside table. African servants brought breakfast, answering, "Yes, madam. No, madam." Elsbeth complimented the couple on their beautiful home and yard. "Oh, but it looks terrible," Mrs. Kunzli responded with a laugh. "Everything is dead. Look at the grass. April is the worst month. There are hardly any flowers left."

Sunday afternoon they sat in the Kunzli's yard playing Swiss music, and all three felt rather homesick. The sky grew darker and darker. In the distance everything was turning brownish yellow. Suddenly the wind started to move small objects on the table. "We'd better go in," Mr. Kunzli said, starting to pick up cups and glasses. Elsbeth watched as the sandstorm moved rapidly across the field, increasing speed and becoming darker and darker brown. Inside the house, she could not see anything but the brown outside the window, could not see the trees in the yard, or the yard itself. All were running like excited children to close the windows. They got to the windows ahead of the storm, but the furniture became coated with the sand anyway, and Elsbeth could feel it crunch between her teeth for hours afterwards.

That evening, at the guest house of the Sudan Interior Mission Language School, Elsbeth hesitated before opening the door to her room. In Switzerland she had gone through a six-month mission course, the first eight weeks of which included a government course on tropical diseases and the insects which carried them. She was used to running from even the smallest spiders, and simply killing a fly was unpleasant for her. The instructors outlined *everything* that could happen and urged all precautions: "Always pick up a toilet seat to see if a scorpion is lurking." "Always wear boots." "Always spray yourself." "Never stand in the sun." "Always have a flashlight." "Always put your mosquito net down."

She wondered, as she opened the door to her room, if there might be any bugs in it. As soon as she turned on the lights, there it was right in the middle of the floor—a huge black insect. *Boy,* she thought, *the troubles of being a single girl! I should have a husband with me. A wife always has her man nearby, even if she sleeps in the bush. He's always ready to kill ugly things like that. Ugh!* She stared at the hideous feelers and slight movements and started pulling off her wooden shoe. She'd never killed anything—but she knew she couldn't sleep with that by her.

Smash!

She got it in one fast whack and immediately felt like a heroine.

But her bug problems were not over. A few nights later she had very carefully tucked her mosquito netting under the mattress. Then she had made a complete tour, going all the way around the bed three times, to make sure no bug could crawl underneath. Finally, she had settled in. Next to her bed was a window through which a bright light from outside came in and lighted her entire room. Relaxing and looking up she saw, right in front of her, a roach which was more than two inches long.

It must be outside the net, Elsbeth thought. *It's one of those big ones that fly.*

But it moved closer and closer, and she realized it was inside with her. Somehow it must have fallen into the net during the day. *If I move, he'll move,* she thought. So, very, very slowly—keeping her eyes exactly on him to make sure she didn't crawl onto him—she worked her way out of the bed. Finally she made it, then walked cautiously to the bathroom to get a heavy bath towel.

Three Countries

She advanced upon the roach. She put the towel over him and smashed him between her two hands.

When she returned the towel to its place by the sink, she thought of the comments friends had made about how roaches come up the drain, and you see the feelers coming up at you. Or you turn on the spigot and *blup,* one falls out into your bathwater.

But the heat was considerably worse than the bugs. Many nights she didn't sleep at all. It made functioning difficult. Once, while observing a cataract operation, she suddenly realized she had to get out of the room. She made it to the hall outside, fainted, lay there for about ten minutes, and then returned to the operating room—unmissed. She had other adjustments. Each morning she would take her malaria pill, shower, then vomit, and lie down. Finally she started taking the pill after drinking four cups of coffee.

The Basel Mission had appointed her to a tiny hospital in Ngoshe, a bush station in the Northeast, by the Cameroon border. The shock of traveling from Zürich to hot, black-African Kano had shoved astonishing impressions into her brain, but the trip to her new home at Ngoshe took her back thousands of years. After an all-night ride by Land-Rover to Maiduguri, she slept a day and visited a leprosarium, then started riding across the flat, beige countryside toward Ngoshe.

Dry. Everything looked dead in the dry season. She grew to appreciate the wispy, twisted trees that broke up the flatness. A few times she would see Africans talking or holding court under a big tree, each man wearing a colorful turban.

Elsbeth rode a hundred bleak miles in the Land-Rover. Just before turning left onto the sixteen-mile road to Ngoshe, a beautiful mountain came into view. It was part of a hundred-mile range; the hospital stood brashly at its base like a flowered, green cactus in a desert. Elsbeth was almost startled by the oasis-green of the hospital compound and the height and mass of the mountain rising above it. Lawns, trees, African flowers. She had anticipated primitive, bleak surroundings and felt refreshed by the *life* which came from the mountain water available here all year long. She was surprised, too, at the nice little house she was shown. It had bedrooms, bath, a guest room, kitchen, and a dining room. The doctor also had a house, and there was a little village for the workers. The doctor had gone to court in Mubi, so his wife, Froda, greeted Elsbeth and served her a lunch of rice and goat meat.

Elsbeth then took a nap, and as soon as she rose asked the nurse, who had just returned from a child-welfare clinic, "May I go see the hospital now?"

The nurse, Maria, smiled. "You will see that soon enough! Why hurry? You'll be sick of it before long." But she took Elsbeth to meet the hospital staff, most of whom spoke only Hausa to her. The hospital had a roofless courtyard inside where patients could sleep on floor mats. On one side were rocks where the patients' relatives could cook food, for the hospital provided none. Inside were fifty-six beds —a male and a female ward, and an eight-bed maternity ward. On the veranda about a hundred sick Africans waited to get into the little dispensary. The women were naked, except for their ornaments; they wore little pearls around their necks or had delicate necklaces and hair ornaments made from fine, wavy strands of grass. The female patients had bones of various sizes—beauty ornaments—hanging through the lower lip. These they used as a toothpick, or ear cleaner, or head scratcher. After use—*blip!*—they would replace it, quick as a turtle blinks, and continue talking with it dangling through the lip. A knob on the end kept it from falling out. The whole place seemed to Elsbeth like a market, with the smell of bean cakes, and yelling and fighting, and flies everywhere.

How can I work here? she wondered. *These conditions!* A woman with a badly infected breast lay behind her. A man on the floor was receiving intravenous fluids. Parents who had lost three children to measles had brought their fourth child—who was almost too far gone. The severity of the medical problems shocked her—they had so little equipment and so small a staff to cope with it all.

She looked into their faces. They smiled. They laughed. They pointed and gestured. The naked children wore amulets around their necks, and the little ones, feathers in their hair, rode in leather skins on the backs of the mothers. Tied to the skins were little calabashes—dried gourds. When the mothers would walk, the red-painted calabashes would make a cute *bloom, bloom, bloom* noise for the child. It became a rattle-type toy for him, but its main function was to keep the evil spirits away.

There had been bugs in Kano. But in Ngoshe, as evening fell and lights were turned on, almost immediately the lamps were full of assorted shapes and movements. Toads were everywhere. She dreaded going into her room alone that first night. Her fingers closed reluctantly on the doorknob. What might be crawling behind it? She eased it open. Nothing was there that she could see, so she walked in and tried to relax. But it wasn't long before she saw something on the wall move fast as a hockey puck. It was orange. Bright orange.

With her eyes, she nailed its location. It was a hairy, ugly spider, about three inches long, shaped like an obese ant with long feelers. *Zoooooom!* It moved again. Elsbeth had never seen anything as fast as that chunky spider. One second he was on the wall, the next he would be on the floor. In fact, where was he now?

She jumped on the bed and screamed, *"Maiguardi! Zo! Zo!"* ("Guard. Come. Come.")

She waited and waited. Finally the guard cautiously opened the door, carefully, carefully, holding his spear at a menacing angle. *"Nama! Nama!"* ("Animal. Animal.")

He advanced ferociously, nimbly like a lion on the hunt, his spear at the ready as Elsbeth tried to explain with her limited Hausa. His bare feet gingerly advanced around the bed as his eyes dug for clues to what might be terrifying the new nurse. A spitting cobra? Elsbeth stood on the bed, not moving, till suddenly she saw the spider on the wall. *"Ka mutu shi! Ka mutu shi!"* ("Die him! Die him!") she screamed.

The spider then zipped onto the floor, and with a casual smack of his foot, the guard demolished the terrorist.

"Huba, Sister!" The guard laughed.

But as jumpy as she was at first, Elsbeth soon found herself adapting. She had been told a little axiom that proved not far from correct: The first year a missionary notices a fly in his tea. He dumps the tea and starts over. The second year he sees a fly and flicks it out, then drinks the tea. The third year he drinks both the fly and the tea! She learned to coexist with all tentacled, hairy, hopping, crawling creatures except one—the chunky, fast-as-a-hockey-puck spider. A regular spider she'd just brush off, but the orange one's speed always frightened her. She grew used to scorpions and snakes. She grew accustomed to the hundreds of lizards which looked like blue, yellow, and red ornaments on the wall. One type she thought looked just like a carrot dunked in ink. Some were as huge as Gila monsters; when one died in the attic, it stank for days.

She grew used to the toads, too. One evening in the rainy season she carefully counted eighty fat ones hopping around in the kitchen. Where did they come from? In the morning they were always gone, but they weren't in the grass, or under the house, or anywhere to be seen. Later she sat down to play the pump organ on the veranda. It wouldn't play—something was wrong. She looked inside, and approximately eighty fat toads returned her stare.

After her first week in Ngoshe, Maria invited Elsbeth to ride in the Land-Rover with her to Barawa, about eight miles away. The blue-purple, rocky hills edged with trees reminded Elsbeth of the vineyards in Germany. Beautiful! Up a hill they went, then pulled into the village. The huts, with their domed tops, looked like tiny Islamic mosques; on top were juju sticks (for charms) resembling feathery crosses poking into the sky.

Elsbeth spied about twenty children, naked, very dirty, and full of flies. Then the villagers came, and they talked for a while. "Well, here is a child for you," Maria observed. "This is Karba." She was touching a two-year-old with a huge belly distended from worms and poor nutrition; the child was so skinny her arms were like sticks. All the hill people had poor diets of Guinea corn every night, rice, and, very seldom, meat—in which case the men ate first. "We could take Karba home for a week," Maria suggested.

"Of course!" Elsbeth agreed. The other nurse knew how much Elsbeth loved children and explained that Karba was an eighth child, which is considered taboo by the hill tribes. They believed that keeping an eighth child would bring disaster on the family and relatives. One tribe would put the baby headfirst into a pot of water to drown it. Another tribe would give these babies to nomads as slaves. The eighth-child tradition was so deep that, even when Christian families kept one and someone got sick or died, it was all the fault of the boy or girl who happened to be born number eight. Relatives with troubles would bitterly blame the Christian family, and the eighth child would feel cursed.

Three Countries

Karba's tribe would dispose of an eighth child by simply putting it out on the rocks to die. Two years before, a Christian chief named Musa had found newborn Karba way up in the mountains of the Druade tribe. He had six children of his own, but he had taken Karba in. But now, Karba needed better nutrition and medical aid.

The two nurses drove Karba back to Ngoshe and stuck her right in the tub. Elsbeth found a leftover crib and some little dresses. She also sewed some underwear for Karba. That first evening they sat her on a pillow to eat, and she used a spoon as if she had always eaten with one. But she was extremely shy and wouldn't talk. "Would you like some more?" Elsbeth coaxed, but Karba stubbornly refused. From the time she had been tiny, she had had to fight for her existence. She was so tough that to Elsbeth it seemed one could almost have killed the two-year-old, and she wouldn't have cried. Yet, in a few days she was happily playing with the doctor's children.

Elsbeth started a baby clinic in Karba's village and went every two weeks with a Nigerian who translated the eight hill-people languages into Hausa. Karba would come running, hug her, and then both would walk in the crowded market. She would keep Karba with her sometimes, especially when she would find her sick and shivering with pneumonia or malaria. Returning Karba was hard for Elsbeth. The little girl would say "Bye-bye" and off she'd go. Five minutes later Elsbeth would see her with a clay pot on her head starting the two-hour trek for water. Elsbeth knew the children accepted Karba fairly well, but there were some who were nasty, because she was an eighth child. When something was stolen, and the natural children would deny it, Karba would get beaten by her stepmother for the misdeed.

Maria and Elsbeth often ran the hospital while Dr. Bakker worked on equipment or drove off on errands. From 100 to 200 patients would be waiting each morning. Elsbeth, who had grown very proficient as a midwife, did the deliveries (including vacuum extractions and suturing). She was in charge of hospital supplies and personnel; yet she often had to take time to drive extreme cases to hospitals which had better equipment. Once, two men who had been fighting with spears were brought in with their intestines hanging out. She rushed them in the Land-Rover over impossibly rutted roads for

110 miles. Arriving at the government hospital, she was told no doctors would be available till after the weekend. She left them there, hoping they'd get attention.

Elsbeth also taught two Sunday-school classes, and language and handicraft classes in her home. Her two-year commitment stretched to three. All the while, Elsbeth was developing a growing love for the genial, fun-loving Africans who could face death and disaster so graciously. *Naked they might be,* she thought, *but in many ways, they are more civilized than we are. They have much to teach us.*

2

Biafra

THE CRANBERRY BOG

Fifteen-year-old David Christensen sat uneasily in his trailer. He had landed a summer job in this New Jersey cranberry bog and was rising to the challenge of construction work and the chance to drive a truck on the muddy lanes. Yet a sense of guilt was making him uneasy. As he undressed on the low fold-down bed, he couldn't evade the memory of his playing the trumpet on Atlantic City's Boardwalk. He always drew a crowd, standing there in the moist air blaring up-temp sounds, and he loved watching the people mill around him to listen. Most of the onlookers didn't realize he was the warmup for an evangelist; but when the preaching started, the crowd quickly melted down to a dozen or so. That was okay with David, but a couple of weeks ago, the evangelist had asked David to speak. Caught off guard, he parroted familiar phrases about how wonderful it was to be a Christian.

Now, as David pulled himself under the covers in the trailer, the words *liar, liar, liar,* taunted his mind and chased away sleep. Hypocrisy. What else was it? He knew he had no personal involvement with God to share with others. Finally he pulled himself out of bed and knelt. He was determined to settle the issue and began to pray.

Nothing happened.

He found himself in a fierce battle. An hour went by, then two. He prayed for salvation, and his praying became more and more intense. "How come if You're there, I don't sense You?" he finally demanded in a near scream. "Where's this fear and guilt coming from? I'm praying. Nothing's happening!"

In the past he had concluded that salvation was all hypocritical nonsense. Now, he wondered if he hadn't been right. But then, at the peak of his cries, he remembered the statement, "For whosoever shall call upon the name of the Lord shall be saved." He thought it all through again: I'm a sinner. I admit it. I repent of my sins. I realize Christ died for me and paid my penalty. I'm calling in the name of Christ and asking Him to come into my heart.

Suddenly David realized something: Who says all this? God says it in His Word, and therefore it's true. On the basis of God's Word, I'm saved!

At that point, everything became different. "Thank You, Lord!" he declared aloud as he experienced a physically tangible sense of peace. "Thank You! Don't ever let me doubt again that You're there!"

The manager of the cranberry bog became ill, and David was left in charge. He felt enormously challenged. One day while driving around the bog in an old car, he slipped off the main track, started to fishtail, and firmly stuck the car in the mud. He then walked a mile to get a farmer who came with a cable and tractor. The farmer promptly pulled the car into a tree, smashing one side severely.

David was mortified. This had been his chance to prove himself as a man! He was determined to show he could cope, so he went around the other way with the truck and aimed at the flimsy board bridge, determined to cross it with utmost care. The tires spread the slats and fell between them; then the weight of the truck made the entire bridge collapse into the water. The truck sank into the mud, crazily tilted half on and half off the bridge.

David surveyed the disaster. How could he face *anyone* now? He was traumatized. He became convinced the only answer was suicide; his death would overshadow the accident, and people would feel sorry for him. But as he looked down at the water, he wondered. Should he drown himself? That would be terribly unpleasant.

Then, almost as if a friend were whispering to him, he heard, "Why don't you pray?"

He dropped to his knees in the water and called out, "God, help me!" Then he walked along in a daze, wondering what to do. As he trudged the New Jersey back road, he passed a parked truck with a road crew in the back. He kept on for almost thirty yards, then abruptly realized, *What have I been praying for?* He scrambled back to the workers and exclaimed to the driver, *"You're the answer to my prayers!*

"Wait a minute! Wait a minute! What is it now?" the man demanded as he tried to calm him down. It took David several minutes to explain his predicament. Finally the entire crew splashed their way into the bog with their crowbars and wedges and started to work on the truck. They pried and blocked and finally pushed it back up the bank. All the men thoroughly enjoyed their Good-Samaritan role. They left David looking at his splattered, cockeyed truck which was now sitting back on the lane.

From then on David walked around the fifty-acre bog. And he reflected on the incident. Was God interested in a fifteen-year-old boy with a truck in the water? David was convinced He was. Not once before, nor once afterward did he ever see a highway crew in the area—let alone one sitting and waiting.

From then on, David was sure of his beliefs. In addition to earning four varsity letters in high school and serving as student council president, he taught Sunday school and was active in a Bible club. In college he led Bible-study sessions and found Inter-Varsity's Urbana Missionary Convention a turning point in his life. Several times he was nearly flabbergasted at the way prayers were remarkably answered. The incidents were too many and too specific to be mere coincidences. He became convinced God was in them.

David needed all this bolstering of his faith for the major testing ahead. By the time he was twenty-two and a medical student, he and his sister Lois, twenty-one, were closer emotionally than ever. They had been the only children in the family, and now as students they went to weddings and other events together. Lois would lend David her car, and David would drive her to the beach. She was the closest person in his life.

Lois joined the Air Force after graduation as an RN, and as she drove to Texas one wet night, her Dodge Dart hydroplaned into a North Carolina ditch and she was killed instantly.

The news of her death jolted David. He was incredulous—just like that, one slide into a ditch, and she was gone forever. It was news too enormous for his mind or emotions to digest.

He talked at her funeral about a grain of wheat needing to fall into the ground and die before it can bear fruit. He mused about her new life in heaven, and wondered what she was doing and thinking now. Yet the vast gulf of separation between him and Lois blocked him from emotions other than grief.

After the funeral he walked alone in the dark and stared at the stars, wondering how God could care and let this happen. Were the stars really linked to God? Or were they white, senseless molecules burning like any trash fire? Were they rubble? Or heavenly gems? What if Lois were dead like a dog? What if she were not conscious anywhere, just extinguished?

He stood under those stars with the fresh weight of Lois's death. No God? But then, where did good come from? And—more pressing —evil? Evil was so horrible, it couldn't be meaningless. All the trails his mind ran down led him back to God and the Bible as the only rational alternative.

MEDICAL STUDENT

David, now twenty-six, was in his last year at Temple University School of Medicine. Each senior could pick an elective. David had chosen to study tropical medicine and, at the same time, to see medical missions firsthand. He was anxious to serve, to plunge in and meet needs, as he visited Sudan Interior Mission hospitals in Nigeria. He looked out the window at the brown, sandy terrain of Galmi. It was 115°. Goats were passing by with colorfully robed Fulani and Hausa herdsmen. As he began sticking his fork into a cold rice salad, a demanding series of knocks interrupted. He opened the door to a virile, muscular young man who was foaming at the mouth, agony contorting his face. The village chief and about sixteen elders crowded around behind him, grimacing and staring as the father excitedly explained the boy had swallowed a needle while sewing.

Galmi, on the edge of the Sahara desert, was the most primitive of the SIM hospitals. Often three patients shared a bed, two on top, one below—then they'd rotate periodically. The operating room was small, yet fairly well equipped. Dr. Jim VerLee had gone to visit several leprosariums, saying to a nurse that David, now a senior medical student, would probably "get baptized by fire."

With everyone crowded around, the baptism had arrived. David attempted to look down the young man's throat. He saw nothing but saliva.

He started the young man toward the operating room, inviting the chief and elders to come and watch. After finding some cocaine, he used an old perfume-spray bottle to anesthetize the boy's throat. Then he probed down with an extra long laryngoscope. The eyes and facial expressions of the chief and elders followed each movement as if the instrument were gagging them as well.

David saw the needle in the esophagus, right below the larynx. His fingers reached for a long, straight hemostat, then lowered it in and grasped the middle of the needle firmly. The boy's father had said the blunt end had been in the mouth, so David figured it had descended first. He pulled gently, cautiously. No good. He increased the tension, trying to free the sharp point. But the needle refused to move.

Mr. Wilf Husband and his wife, Esther, stepped into the operating room. They wondered how the young "doctor" was getting along and suggested they pray. Everyone nodded approval, and David agreed. After the prayer, with everyone anxiously watching him, he felt the almost physical pressure and tension of the room. If he vigorously tried to free the blunt end of the needle, he might puncture the spinal cord with the sharp point. He would risk vocal cord damage in the other direction.

Opting for the latter, he slowly pushed the blunt tip through the trachea until there was a bulge in the skin. Then he carefully scrubbed and draped the boy's neck. With the chief and elders straining forward to watch, he made an incision. Then with sterile forceps, he pulled at the needle.

David watched the young man's apprehension fade as the three-inch needle slowly came out. He held it in the air. The spectators' faces brightened as the operating room exploded with Hausa and English exclamations of joy and congratulations.

"Please give me the needle," the chief asked.

"No," David replied. "I would like to keep it as my payment."

The chief and elders all expressed their approval. David returned to his supper feeling like a conquering hero. In fact, he felt as if he'd just been awarded his M.D. He'd been able to think and remain cool under pressure. A life had been saved.

But that evening, a young girl from miles away was brought in, having been bitten severely by a horse, and he had no time for drifting on hero's clouds. Medicine in Africa is far more often serious emergency care than it is in the States. Tribesmen do not go to doctors for checkups. They come when they haven't eaten properly for three months due to pyloric scarring.

When David had first planned a trip to Galmi, he had expected an unpleasant experience. It was said to be dry, desolate, and discouraging. Everything was primitive. Missionaries had to sacrifice—Dave pictured Dr. VerLee as an emaciated martyr with bags under his eyes. He was surprised when he arrived to see fairly nice homes—some with gardens, crops, and chickens. A generator, a windmill, and a well provided electricity, running water, toilets, and showers. He experienced, as the days went by, a delight in the African people.

David had arrived in Kano, Nigeria, in January 1967. He was met by the harmattan, a rain of dust thick enough to delay his flight to Jos. He came on the heels of the massacres of Ibo tribesmen just two months before, and as he walked around the Kano airport he had seen the places where the initial tribal-hatred atrocities had occurred. He had read about them in *Time* magazine:

A Lagos-bound BOAC jet had just arrived from London, and as the Kano passengers were escorted into the customs shed a wild-eyed soldier stormed in, brandishing a rifle and demanding *"Ina Nyamiri"*—Hausa for "Where are the damned Ibos?" There were Ibos among the customs officers, and they dropped their chalk and fled, only to be shot down in the main terminal by other soldiers. The Hausa troops turned the airport into a shambles, bayonetting Ibo workers in the bar, gunning them down in the corridors, and hauling Ibo passengers off the plane to be lined up and shot.

(October 7, 1966)

David was driven to the market in Kano, where women of many tribes, dressed in brightly colored cloth, had pounded pepper and corn. Now the tin huts and booths were deserted. "This house is where a whole family was murdered," he was told as they drove past ruined homes.

Next day David flew to Jos where he talked to the missionary dentist. Weeks before, his houseboy had jumped screaming into the dentist's arms, but Hausas had slashed the Ibo boy to death. Men, women, and children had been shot, stabbed, or burned to death. Pregnant women had been slashed open. Almost two million had fled from the North. Over thirty thousand Easterners—Ibos, Efiks, Ijaws, Ibibios, Ogojas—had been murdered.

It was hard for David to comprehend all this. But as he traveled to hospitals in Nigeria and read and evaluated, he glimpsed a complex set of causes based on tribal loyalties, ancient hatreds, colonialistic absurdities, and the terrible price of making a nation of tribes which for centuries had been mortal enemies.

Yet the massacres were past. What dug into his emotions most deeply were the human needs he saw around him. David drove sixty miles over dirt roads from Egbe to the town of Patigi on the Niger River. There a nurse in her late fifties, Nancy Cairns, cared for sixty patients. When David arrived she had delivered thirty-four babies in the past fourteen days—five the night before his arrival. Sixteen mothers were ready to deliver. There were only eight beds in the maternity building, so eight mothers were on the floor. Twenty mothers with infants were in another small building, many of them on the floor. Another building held twenty seriously ill patients. Nurse Cairns also saw outpatients every morning and lepers several days a week in another location. There was no doctor for sixty miles. David felt depressed in the extreme humidity. *If this sickly, older woman can do all this in such oppressive heat, why can't I?* The experience made him willing to return, regardless of unpleasantness.

In Africa David experienced surprise at how filth mixed with beauty and failures contrasted with achievement. He was full of enthusiasm as he assisted in operations and diagnostic work. He wrote home:

Last Thursday Dr. Dion Warren and I went over the dirt roads for forty miles to one of the SIM leprosariums. Over 100 disfigured lepers; what a sobering experience! A full-time doctor should be correcting dropped feet, operating on osteomyelitis, repairing faces . . . .

The various physical problems are indescribable—a six-month waiting list for people who need surgery here at Egbe.

So much to do. So much left undone. It's hard to just stop around seven o'clock when there are very ill patients who have traveled many miles and have not even been seen by a nurse all day. Yet allowing myself to work around the clock would make me tired and soon useless. Besides, many evenings I'm in the operating room assisting on strangulated hernias, C-sections and other emergencies. Two patients have died, but we've done much good for many.

Egbe is a wonderful village, miles from civilization. The missionaries are really in love with the Lord. The first night I attended a compound prayer meeting with about twenty missionaries. There was a tremendous spirit of kinship and meaningful prayer and praise.

There are two churches in Egbe, one with a congregation of 600, the other with 400. You should hear them sing! I've had Bible study and prayer with some of the Africans, and they have much to teach me.

They're friendly. They love to greet you and always curtsy when they start to talk or when they pass you on the road. They love to laugh. And they're noisy. I can often hear two of them conversing a quarter mile away. They shout to each other.

This tribe's language, Yoruba, is very musical. The tone and pitch change the meaning. For instance, if they sing the chorus "He Lives" to our tune, it would mean "He laid an egg."

The people here are somewhat cleaner than up North. But their houses —ramshackle mud huts—are not like the pretty northern huts with their straw-thatched roofs. Their clothes are robe-type affairs often draped on without underclothes—cool and practical. They eat mostly yams—awful, black, paste-like stuff they eat out of a bowl with their fingers.

Of course, there is still paganism and idol worship. There was a human sacrifice near here just recently.

WAR ZONE

By the time David returned to Nigeria as an SIM doctor a year and a half later, Biafra had seceded and the civil war had begun. The world was starting to see photos of starving Biafran children, and the horrors of war were exceeding those of the massacres before it. Atrocities and "just causes" enflamed the emotions of both sides.

By late spring of 1969, Biafra was shrinking into a smaller and smaller chunk of the East. Port Harcourt, formerly an Ibo town, had been seized by the Nigerian government and David was asked to join a medical relief team. He arrived on a small Nigerian Airways plane to see Port Harcourt widely gutted. The Biafrans had burned the big department stores as they had left. Cars were stranded along the potholed, bombed roads. Houses and huts looked like a series of hurricane-disaster photos. Yet David was impressed that the Nigerian army had resisted massacring the people. The soldiers had watched as ninety thousand Ibos had evacuated the city in one night.

Now, the Ogoni river people had entered Port Harcourt. But they had been subjugated by the Ibos for so long, they didn't know how to run it. The city lay like a smashed clay pot. Treated like America's "niggers," the Ogonis had not even been allowed on the elevators in Port Harcourt, let alone permitted in the schools. When David arrived at the Bori hospital forty miles southeast of Port Harcourt, he found by the medical records that almost everyone operated on had been Ibo, that only in extreme circumstances would an Ogoni be treated, and then he would be charged outrageous prices. All were government doctors who were supposed to charge nothing, yet right under David's hand were the financial records showing immense profits. Recently, hundreds of Ibo doctors, nurses, and patients had been killed in revenge.

David's initial work was providing general care in the 120-bed Bori hospital. In addition, his big specialty became hernias. It seemed everyone had hernias, huge basketball-size ones. To complicate matters, the Ogonis had a taboo against hernias—one could not be buried in his village if he had one. Daily, as David entered his office there was a mad rush, accompanied by all the sounds of a riot. The patients marched in, hobbling, limping, wincing, and contorting, trying to convince the doctor their case was very special. When put on a waiting list, they pled, argued, looked mournful, and refused to leave the room. They wanted immediate action, insisting it was indecent to be seen in public with such large hernias.

The hospital soon flourished. David conducted his "hernia repair factory" with a miner's-type flashlight on his head, repairing sixty hernias in three weeks. He treated hundreds of outpatients. At dusk, David would hear Biafran-relief planes flying overhead as the sun went down, and he could hear shooting in the Northeast.

Once a Russian-made MIG flew in low overhead. Instantly nurses, patients, and soldiers dived out of the windows. It reminded David of walking into a room full of roaches and stamping his feet—*poof,* the hospital was empty. Only one patient remained in the entire hospital—a man wrapped in casts. Outside, seriously ill patients lay flat in the grass near belly-down medical personnel. David couldn't see one of them. These people had been through war and knew how to disappear.

The war continued, but David had to leave Bori to return to Jos. He stayed at a Port Harcourt hotel on the way. In the morning as he arose, he noticed the dawn. Cool air was fresh and sweet as a brilliantly golden sun appeared over the horizon. It was a bright, exhilarating morning. There was scarcely a cloud in the sky. Yet as he looked toward the tropical forest, he was horrified. The sky was filled with vultures. They were circling the site of the Port Harcourt hospital. He was used to seeing three or four of the scavengers lazily floating in search of carrion; but there, in a vertical-cone formation, were literally hundreds of them—like bombers in a blitz in World War II.

Then he realized what they were after. A new shipment of wounded and dying soldiers had just been brought from the front. The vultures were slowly, expectantly circling the hospital in graceful formation, like a cloud of death above the soldiers.

What in the world was God doing? Massacres of whole families! Prejudice and graft, killings and hatred, starving children and tortured students—vultures above all humanity! What sort of world had God dumped him into? He watched the vultures in the bright, warming air. If God was omnipotent, how could He allow all this and not be the author of evil? Man can do nothing unless God lets him—why blame man for all this hatred and carnage?

Who was God? What was He like? David thought for a long while. The Book of James said God never does wrong or tempts anyone to sin. And Habakkuk said God's pure eyes can't look on iniquity. God was good. All good. So good He even went to the extreme of allowing evil to exist because in some strange way, far beyond David's immediate view, all the devastation and pain would someday bring joy.

No, David thought, *God was not the author of evil. He had given man the chance to obey or disobey, to choose good or evil. Man's choice was obvious.*

My own love is so small. He remembered Jesus' statement that the greatest commandments were: "Thou shalt love the Lord thy God with all thy heart, and with all thy soul, and with all thy mind," and "Thou shalt love thy neighbor as thyself." *If we were acting on Jesus' words,* David thought, *this war would not be happening.*

3

Two Weeks in the Bush

ROUGH ROAD

By January 1970 the civil war was over, and David found himself driving an old Volkswagen from Jos to a little village far North named Ngoshe. A few weeks before he had befriended two women he'd met in a bookstore—Froda Bakker and Elsbeth Zurbüchen, a black-haired nurse who was about his age. The women had run into trouble getting their VW fixed in Jos. Parts had been delayed, and they would have to return. David had offered to wait for the parts, then take his vacation and drive the VW to Ngoshe for them—provided they would join him in visiting the Wasa Game Reserve.

As he left Evangel Hospital, Administrator Joan Potter cautioned, "Make sure you don't fall in love with some—with that nice Swiss girl up there."

"Don't worry about that," David responded. Actually he expected Elsbeth to be gone. She had by now served three years in Ngoshe and had been due to fly back to Switzerland almost two weeks before. He considered Elsbeth an unusually attractive friend but had no strongly romantic thoughts.

After about ten hours of driving, he aimed the VW into the deep ruts of the road from Maiduguri to Ngoshe. The roadbed was built far up over swampland. He felt as if he were driving precariously on top of a narrow dam without protective railings. Big trucks would roar down upon him, and David would grimace with thoughts of drivers killed on roads like this.

After a couple hours, he found the little Ngoshe sign and turned toward the mountains. He drove past brown and gray brush and trees shriveled into odd shapes, at times having to bounce through gullies where bridges had been washed out. After sixteen miles, he saw a Hospital sign hammered onto a tree. He turned onto the dirt road piled with sand and, after a few minutes, arrived at a gate with metal pipes across it to keep the goats out. The mountain before him was stone—with boulders jutting out like small houses. The road ended in a circle, and as he emerged thirsty and cramped, the doctor's children ran toward him, then Froda came to greet him.

Elsbeth heard him arrive as she sat sipping lemonade with Maya, the new nurse. They had looked through the openings in the stone wall, and Maya had taunted, "There's your doctor!" Maya had left to greet him, but Elsbeth had no intention of joining her. Staff members had teased her about "her doctor," especially when David had sent a telegram—"parts still not available"—addressed to her instead of Froda. "Uh huh, uh huh, a single doctor, eh?" And one day in Jos David had stiffened her resolve to show no romantic interest! She and Froda had stopped at his house to say good-bye and he had invited them in for dinner. They hadn't expected much at a bachelor's home, but Anthony the cook had served them royally. David had befriended them numerous times during the past week and he had wanted them to know he wasn't fishing for anything. He had abruptly announced at the dinner table, "I want you to understand that I'm not doing any of this for some ulterior purpose." Fire had lighted in Elsbeth's eyes. *Huh! So that's the way he feels. Boy, he'll never get the impression I'm after him. Does he feel he is the important, uncatchable rooster and girls the lowly hens? No one is ever going to think, in any way—especially not you, Doctor David Christensen—that I am hoping I might be the privileged one!*

But Froda brought David over to Elsbeth's house and asked, "Why don't you take David along on your walk?" Elsbeth had to visit a woman in the next village about three miles away. "I suppose that would be all right," Elsbeth responded evenly.

David soon found himself climbing up and down rocks behind Elsbeth as she picked her way along a footpath. Birds sang, rustled, and flew away. Goats clattered off at the sight of them. They stopped at some huts which were surrounded by a wall of matted brush and thorn bushes to keep the goats out. The husband and each wife had separate huts. *"Usa! Usa!"* Elsbeth greeted. *"Usa! Sister!"* they responded.

David watched Elsbeth warmly converse about babies, grandmothers, and children, with laughter often bubbling out. Elsbeth kept turning to David to explain the conversation. Her natural, subtle humor about the harvest and rainy season and the moon and corn interested and amused the villagers. Elsbeth's eyes danced, and her smile had an intelligence linked beautifully to her eyes. David was grateful that she pulled him into the circle and made him feel included.

It was getting dark. They hurried on. Despite Elsbeth's warmth, concern, and openness, she gave him no reason to think that there might be any special magic between them. She acted like a friendly tour guide in the Swiss Alps, a lively conversationalist who would smile when appropriate, and one to whom he would pay ten francs after the walk. But as he watched her ahead of him, he admired her gutsiness in coming out to a place like this. He had visited bush stations before, but this was isolation. The nearest place to buy supplies was a hundred miles away. Yes, she was gutsy. And attractive, with her long, dark hair styled in a typical Swiss bun. She walked with a strut that was very determined, yet feminine.

At the next mission compound, they walked up to the house and knocked. David was shocked at the woman who answered. Her face and arms were scarred from major burns, but it was her anger that made her look ghastly. She crackled flames of indignation at Elsbeth about dinner guests who had cancelled on her. David stood there a bit awkwardly as the two women conversed in German. Elsbeth's soft answers and poise drew the anger out of the woman. He saw her emotions subsiding and observed how Elsbeth the peacemaker did not get caught up in the conflict. *What class!* he thought. *Now here's a mature woman who knows how to handle people.*

They returned to the hospital compound but found that Nieck, Froda's husband, was still too sick to even say hello. This meant Elsbeth and Maya would not be able to go with David to the game

BARAWA BABY CLINIC

Elsbeth had made a decision in the last few weeks, and it had not come easily. Her commitment to Ngoshe was over. Her plane tickets had been delayed in Kano, but she was to leave in a few days. She had grown to deeply love the people, and the needs were enormous. Yet her decision would probably set her direction for life. If she returned to Africa, she would probably never get married. She loved children and wanted her own; and if she stayed in Switzerland, she might find the right man.

She had had opportunities to marry. A Britisher she had met in Kano had come to Ngoshe numerous times and had proposed to her. Back in Switzerland was Rolf, who loved her very much. A physicist and astronomer, Rolf had taken six months off work to build her a Morse code transmitter so she could contact Berne from Nigeria. Because of the Biafran war, they wouldn't let it into the country. When Elsbeth told Rolf of the problem, he had said, "That's all right, whatever they decide. I learned a lot and I'll be able to use it somehow." He was a "fourth brother" to her and a wonderful friend.

But she had determined she would never marry just for the sake of marrying and for children, no matter how much she wanted them. She was an intensely sexual person with very strong drives, yet she had to have a man she could genuinely, deeply love. After Claus, she doubted she could again. "Lord, You know me," she had prayed a few weeks ago. "You know how I am made. I want to get married. You have to show me." As she prayed, Jesus' words, "Seek ye first the kingdom of God and all these things will be added unto you," became dominant in her mind. She made her decision to return to Ngoshe. As soon as she did, she immediately felt free, gloriously free, and ready to come back after her trip to Switzerland.

So, as she hurriedly cared for outpatients early Friday morning, she had no thought of romance—and that certainly included this

Two Weeks in the Bush

single-doctor tagalong. Even now he was following her, watching procedures. She was just days away from flying home. Nieck was ill. She was ruthlessly rushed.

Froda had asked yesterday, "Elsbeth, aren't you going to Barawa tomorrow?"

"Yes."

Then Froda had turned to David. "Wouldn't you be interested in going out there? It is a nice village." So what could Elsbeth say? She had to let him come along.

They walked out to the Land-Rover. David had been impressed with the way Elsbeth ran the hospital and did a doctor's job. She was an interesting person and a bit of a challenge to his male ego. However, instead of a friendly twosome, into the Land-Rover went a translator, two girl assistants, a table, two chairs, a bag of drugs, two big containers of water, a can of gas, and a basket of food. David was kindly, but pointedly, shown a seat in the back; and there he sat, crammed in with the supplies.

Rrroar!! Elsbeth ripped off in the jam-packed Land-Rover at what felt like sixty mph. David was jerked back and thought that if he had been wearing false teeth they would have been in his throat. Yet he was amazed to see Elsbeth's way with the rough, trucklike vehicle. She dodged the potholes expertly and wheeled her way through the ruts and streams. After eight miles she stopped at a collection of huts at the foot of the mountains. On an open plain David could see people gathering under a big tree. It was eight in the morning and already getting hot.

Karba, as soon as she heard the Land-Rover, was the first to come running up to Elsbeth. They hugged and kissed and Karba stuck close to her "Mommy." The staff set up the table under the tree. Before long hundreds of people from miles away had gathered, all eager to trade at the village market. Mothers would drop over to the clinic, and Elsbeth would weigh the babies, check their records, and give them milk, vaccinations, and medicine. She had started this clinic herself with just a few children. Today, there would be sixty-six children with runny noses, hundreds of rainy-season flies on their faces, and distended stomachs. Elsbeth knew all the mothers by name. Several chiefs from various villages in the mountains stopped by to greet her.

David explored the market. He waited a half hour to photograph an old man in just the right position in front of his hut. By the time he'd snapped two rolls of film and returned, Elsbeth was still not done. He sat patiently focusing on Elsbeth, carefully getting the proper angle, looking for the right expression—then she'd notice him and snap her head the other way. He moved and tried again. She spied him and moved her chair.

Despite the rebuff, David was impressed with the way she was always making the Africans laugh. Her timing was perfect; she'd slip in a word or phrase at just the right moment and the villagers would explode with laughter. Elsbeth was constantly talking up the bright side. She coped with difficulties, lovingly yet firmly. Little sand flies were biting viciously, and each child had literally scores of flies resting around both eyes, but it did no good to shoo them. They were so thick, David saw one go right down Elsbeth's throat.

Once in a while Elsbeth would ask what he thought of a patient with malarial or other serious symptoms. She told him that one day a mother had brought a child with a foot so far gone that Elsbeth had simply taken it off with her hand. The bone had stuck out a little and she had dressed it; later it had healed.

The activities died down a bit, and Elsbeth took a break. They all climbed into the Land-Rover. A bowl of *kuno* (a sour porridge made from rice) with *tsamia* (a lemonlike fruit) was passed around. The translator and staff girls and David and Elsbeth ate with a common spoon. The flies were all over the food in black clumps. They ate *kosse* (fried bean cakes with salt and pepper) and goat meat. They passed around a thermos of tea, and David sensed they were all having a bit of fun with him, realizing he wasn't used to all this. Elsbeth ignored David and expertly dipped three fingers into the heavy Guinea corn porridge, scooped gravy onto it and ate. She acted oblivious to any idea this was not typical behavior. David gamely ate one mouthful of the *kuno*. It was a mistake—he didn't have the "antibodies" the others did and later he would become ill.

Elsbeth got down from the Land-Rover and was immediately jammed into the crowds again. She had to watch where she placed

Two Weeks in the Bush

her feet so she wouldn't step on a child. She would never forget how terrifying a crowd of people like this could be if they panicked. During the war she had noticed a policeman riding around this market on a horse. Suddenly it had started stomping, whinnying, and going out of control. Within seconds a thousand people had panicked. Those in the middle had been crushed. Another day she had been sitting under this same tree with about forty-five women waiting with their children. Horns and loudspeakers had brashly interrupted: NO ONE IS ALLOWED TO MOVE FROM THE MARKET! Of course, that had been the worst thing they could have announced. The women had grabbed children with one arm, swinging them up onto their backs and scrambling up the stones like goats. Everywhere naked bodies had scattered as a dozen policemen with weapons had run after them. They had caught some of the women with children and had dragged them back. Other policemen had organized their "shotguns" for measles and smallpox vaccinations. Each child had gotten one in both arms. Some of the women had then run away again and they had been dragged back again. The policemen hadn't bothered to ask or listen—they "shot" these children twice! In four minutes the marketplace had become completely empty. Elsbeth had sat alone with her cards and medicines, furious. The fleeing mothers were far up in the mountains, each wearing only a fur on her back to hold her child, jumping from one rock to the other, up, up, up. It was a five-hour climb to the top where Karba was born, but they would clamber up in a half hour.

She and David now walked among the people and looked at the village church—a big hut with domed top and a cross poking into the sky. David looked at it closely. *We think our civilization is so great,* he thought. *But look at all those stones put together without mortar.* He looked up at the hills where the trees edged around the rocks like thick moss. About ten thousand hill people lived up there; not one of their languages was on paper yet. On coming to market, they'd carry colorful cloths to wrap around them when they arrived, but only because it was the law to wear clothes. They were naked. They worshiped ancestors. They sacrificed goats and cows. Yet they had so much to teach about endurance, fortitude, and simplicity.

Five hours had passed. It was time to load the Land-Rover. A half-dozen sick people were to go back, including Karba, who had pneumonia. Since patients had to provide their own food, big sacks of Guinea corn and filled calabashes were tossed in, with the people impossibly jammed around them. Of course, David had to find a few inches in the middle of all this. It was 112°; the Land-Rover was a closed vehicle; and the people were not only full of flies but, judging from the smell, they were utterly unwashed. Leaves of dried grass on their open sores did nothing to dissuade the flies, and David wondered if he could survive the stench. Elsbeth took off with a roar again, dodging holes and ruts as babies cried and children shrieked. These people had never been in a car before. David looked over at Karba, her face white with dirt. She had a distended belly, cough, runny nose, flies, and lice. He marveled at Elsbeth's love for the girl.

David was very glad to get a shower after Barawa. He saw some patients and then he rested. The game reserve plans were shot for now, and if he wanted to see it, he would have to stay several more days. He read *The Autobiography of Malcolm X* and the Book of Proverbs, where he found a number of helpful statements—including some intriguing ones about how a man falls in love with a woman. In late afternoon he stepped out and sat under a tree by a little flower garden and found that Dr. Bakker—Nieck—was a little better. Elsbeth came over for a while, and after she left, David found himself asking Nieck his opinions about falling in love. "Now take Elsbeth, for instance," he conjectured. "Here's a nice girl, somebody I admire. But how would one know if he's in love with someone like that?"

MUBI

Elsbeth knocked on David's window at six o'clock Wednesday morning. "Dave, we should leave." He was sound asleep; but as soon as her voice got through to him, he was up instantly, feeling like a little boy being called by Mother. He hated to be late for anything. After yanking and pulling on his clothes, he was outside in minutes. They had agreed the night before to leave at six. He skipped breakfast and strode out to the VW.

Mubi was about a hundred miles away, but Elsbeth didn't bother

Two Weeks in the Bush

to tell him. At first Elsbeth had planned to go alone, but Froda had asked, "Aren't you taking Dave with you?"

"No."

"Why? Wouldn't it be nice to have company?"

"Well, yes, I guess so," and Elsbeth had realized she didn't very much enjoy driving the rough roads. She had assented, and Froda had invited David.

During the past few days, David had become increasingly intrigued with Elsbeth. Saturday evening he had watched her relate to Froda and Nieck. She was a marvelous storyteller, illustrating her tales of the day with appropriate grunts, *hoomphs,* and gestures. And such a smile Elsbeth had! They had all listened to classical music, and they had also brought a musician in from the hills. All bone and muscle and wearing only a fur, the man had never been in a white man's building before. He had played an *nrule,* a C-shaped instrument. It was made from a Guinea corn stick which was covered with goat skin, and wire strings were attached. Each finger touched a string as the man told tribal stories in what sounded like an Arabic chant. He had been melodic and fascinating, and David had watched Elsbeth's enthusiastic appreciation. Everywhere they went, David noticed her deep love for the Nigerians.

The road to Mubi was rough and unfamiliar to David, who was trying to make good time on it. They stopped very briefly at an old house at Gulak to greet some missionaries, Doeke and Sjoerdtje Land. They were friendly to Dave, but they spoke German, so he went off to play with the children as Elsbeth talked. He was not aware that Sjoerdtje commented to Elsbeth, "Oh, you have company today? A young doctor? Can we congratulate?" The words reminded her of the way people viewed their being together. Elsbeth assured the woman very clearly that no congratulations were in order.

They went on to Mubi, where they visited the Scheytts who helped to run a Bible school. All students learned farming, and when graduates would go into the villages, they took both the Gospel and commonsense farm methods with them. Wilhelm Scheytt, a German, had been in Nigeria eleven years and was field superintendent of Basel Mission. He had written books and Bible courses and had formed an orchestra to play indigenous music. Wilhelm and Elsbeth went to the police station to fill out papers, while David relaxed at their home. "An unusual girl, that Elsbeth," Martha Scheytt commented to him after they'd left. "Very capable and deep. Beautiful, too." David agreed with her.

After lunch, Elsbeth, Wilhelm, and David went to a marketplace. Elsbeth was looking for gifts to take back to Switzerland. They evaluated a brass money-holder with leather strings and little bells which showed impressive workmanship. They also looked over "dinner" bells. David inspected some and finally picked out one he liked. Wilhelm started to help David bargain for the little gleaming bell, but before he could buy it, Elsbeth snatched it from David's hand, saying, "This is the bell I wanted to buy." Her motive was to give it to David later as a token of appreciation for his kindnesses, but he didn't know that. He felt confused.

Well, that was going to change! He started to feel aggressive. Wilhelm and Elsbeth were now making a big fuss over some brass ornaments. Although he saw no value in them, and they seemed overpriced, when Elsbeth picked one out he moved right in and declared, "Here, I'm going to pay for that."

"Oh, no!!!" Elsbeth retorted immediately.

But David was determined. He insisted on buying one for himself and one for Elsbeth, who bristled. Her attitude of stern disapproval was in no way softened when Wilhelm whispered into her ear in German, "That's the way it starts." The comment nearly made her storm out of the market. She liked and admired David. But if others saw something between them, perhaps something was there. She couldn't allow those thoughts, so she insisted on a rigidly platonic friendship.

Later the two couples ate dinner, and David sensed the romantic electricity growing between him and Elsbeth. It seemed natural that they were relating here as a couple. He sensed the challenge, but he wasn't quite sure what to do about it. Should he give in to the feelings growing in him? Was it merely his male ego asserting itself? She was leaving the country—was it realistic to allow these feelings to grow?

Elsbeth was still strictly courteous and correct with him, and Martha's farewell after supper did nothing to push her closer to

Two Weeks in the Bush

David. "Bye-bye, Elsbeth," she called out in Swiss German as they drove off. "See you in August, either single or married!"

They drove with Elsbeth decidedly on her side of the car, talking appreciatively about the Scheytts. Eventually the subject turned to nurses, and David made one of the larger mistakes of the day by launching into a speech about nurses' shortcomings. He felt that generally they were nonthinking, did not take initiative, and let themselves be walked on too much. He went on and on, and as a windup to his observations, he commented, "Of course, Elsbeth, you are an exception."

"I am an exception!" she exploded. "Why should I be an exception? You don't have to say that just to make me feel good. I'm *not* an exception. I am a nurse. I can't stand it when people tell a long story and explain everything they hate; and then they say, kindly and sweetly, 'Oh, but *you* are an exception.' " Now it was her turn to go on and on.

Oh, no, he thought. *Here we are, finally alone, relating and talking civilly, and now this!* "I can't judge everybody," he answered a bit lamely. "I'm just saying that's my overall impression. It depends on a nurse's training and . . . ."

She rebutted his excuses effectively, and David thought, *Every young man has a speech about something. Why did this have to be mine!* But he wasn't sure she was really angry. He thought he saw a twinkle of humor in all that fire. Coming back from the Barawa market a few days ago she had been declaring she would never marry an American, she would never go to the States where everything was oriented to money and modern machines and there was no culture, and she would *certainly never marry a doctor!* He sensed she liked to tease him, and he hoped her rich vein of humor was providing most of the fireworks now. He liked the fact that she was his intellectual match.

As they pulled into the mile-long sand road leading to the hospital, Elsbeth began to feel it was a shame they had argued so much. She enjoyed his company and the verbal combat, but now she wanted to let him know she was really not that angry. As they drove past the gate and into the dark compound, David said, "I don't know how to put it, but . . . ."

Elsbeth gulped, wondering, *Oh no, what is he going to say now?* "I enjoyed this day very, very much," he faltered. "I've enjoyed being with you. I don't know how to express this—I don't know how it's possible—but one thing I know, I want to get to know you better. I'm in God's hands, you're in God's hands. God knows His choice for me. I ask you to pray about it as I am praying about it."

From that evening on, everything was changed between them. They could no longer be just friends. The old relationship was over—Elsbeth feared he would pick up that conversation again, so she avoided him. David tried to sort out his feelings. By Monday she'd be gone. His attentions were being rebuffed, yet he felt drawn to her. Was God trying to tell him something from all the coincidences? Again and again in Jos, circumstances had pulled them together. And now his short stay was stretching to two weeks—and the hospital administrator had said before he left, "Why not take two weeks?"

He was determined to be objective. He even started a list of pros and cons about Elsbeth. *Con:* Indecisive at times. *Pro:* She drove all the way from Jos to Ngoshe in a jeep—she's persistent and capable. *Pro:* Attractive? Definitely! *Pro:* Spiritual depth.

He was concerned primarily about one thing—trusting God, and looking for His leadership. He thought back to a day shortly after his sister Lois had been killed. He had been dating a girl named Carol and getting rather serious about her. But then he had seen her in church with a student named Mike, and he had sensed by her expression that she loved Mike. Yet David also knew she had deep affection for him. What should he do? For a full ten minutes he had battled the questions in his mind. Should he fight for Carol? He felt he had a good chance of winning. *But if I really love her,* he had thought, *don't I put her first? Just because I feel love, does that mean I grab her? If Carol will be happier with Mike, shouldn't I give her to him?* He had prayed that God would help him with his emotions, and he felt clearly led to give Carol up. After that he had become a close friend of Mike's; he had concluded that, in any situation, one can act out of self-interest or one can seek God's plan.

It was surely that way here. Were all these coincidences blending with biblical principles and his own feelings about Elsbeth in a way that said, "She's the one for you"? Was God behind all this? He wanted to know that above all else.

If only he had more than a few days to come to a conclusion!

BIRTH

The next morning Froda was talking to David about various subjects and then indicated that Nieck needed his help in the hospital. "The sisters are very upset. In fact," Froda added with an impish smile, "you might see Elsbeth in a different light this time."

"Well, I don't want to interfere," David admitted.

"Yes, but I think Nieck needs your support. What do you think of symphysiotomies?"

David had never done one, but he was familiar with the procedure from the medical books. Instead of a Caesarean at a difficult birth, the doctor would cut the ligaments at the midline of the pubic bone. The severing would give the baby an extra inch or so to get his head through. "With careful selection of cases, it's a sound, approved procedure," David assured her. Froda then persuaded him to walk down to assist.

However, as he poked his head rather sheepishly into the operating room, he was immediately confronted by Elsbeth's angry eyes. They looked like black daggers which would have jabbed him out of the room. She was opening packs of cotton and medicine for the expected baby and forced a grunt of hello. Nieck, bearded and rugged-looking, yet trembling, greeted him cordially.

That's all I need, Elsbeth thought to herself. She had already been angry, and now David had to walk in. She felt like grabbing him by the neck and pitching him out the door, especially when Nieck in an overly friendly manner started explaining his plans. His African assistant looked on. Elsbeth and Maya had told Nieck they would refuse to assist on another symphysiotomy. But at the last minute Elsbeth had decided to come in for the sake of the baby and mother. In the time Elsbeth had been at Ngoshe, Nieck had done about five Caesarean sections, all successful. However, there was a lack of blood, oxygen, and lab support in the bush, and he had lost C-section patients previously. So he started doing the symphysiotomies. One woman had died. But Elsbeth and Maya's most volatile objection was that he didn't numb the pain sufficiently. The women had suffered terribly.

David, of course, knew none of this, except that Elsbeth was angry and banging utensils and bottles. He was shocked, for previously she had exuded love and warmth and fun. He began discussing with Nieck the key steps of the procedure and realized Nieck had probably missed some of them on previous occasions. Nieck inserted a needle to numb the area. As he started to cut through to the bone, the woman cried out. "Why don't you use a long needle?" David suggested. Nieck injected more painkiller, then cut through the ligaments just enough to spread the bone. The woman had been pushing all this time, and as soon as the bone gave way they could see the baby's head coming. In five minutes it was born. It was white because of the stress on the head. Nieck now had to stop the bleeding in the mother and deliver the placenta.

It was fortunate Elsbeth had come. The baby wasn't breathing. Its mouth and throat were full of mucus and she had to suck it out with a tube and give mouth-to-mouth resuscitation for fifteen minutes. She injected Coramine; she slapped him; finally the baby came around.

When the baby had perked up, David felt rather useless standing around, so he walked back to the Bakker house. Froda had lunch nearly ready and asked, "How was it?"

"I think it went very well," David responded. "Everything's fine." He grinned a bit and added, "You know what, Froda? Elsbeth was furious. And I found out I even like her when she's mad. She's even more beautiful when she's angry."

WASA GAME RESERVE

At noon Friday David gripped the very loose steering wheel of the Land-Rover and started off with Maya, Elsbeth, and Karba, who had recovered from her pneumonia. He felt a bit clumsy as he tried to dodge potholes. They crossed a riverbed and then the Cameroon border. The road to the game reserve was sandy, which threw the Land-Rover right and left as David fought to stay in the tracks left by other

Two Weeks in the Bush

vehicles. Around three o'clock they pulled up to the registration office and Elsbeth, who had told David she didn't really speak French, fluently interacted with the registrar. The fenced-in compound was located on a hill, higher than the game reserve and about a half hour's drive from it. At the very top of the hill was a restaurant.

David had trouble getting the Land-Rover up the steep grade to their rented hut. After showering, they hired an African guide and drove across the flat bushland with its sections of oddly twisted trees. Everything in the distance was brownish yellow, so the animals were well hidden. Yet Karba's sharp eyes would spot the animals before the guide could. They would drive as close to the animals as possible, jam on the brakes, and everyone would run out to take pictures.

Elsbeth began having trouble with her camera's battery. David worked to fix it and realized a bad connection ran down the batteries, so he'd remove them between each shot. At first Elsbeth didn't want him helping, but then as he fixed it each time, she realized their teamwork was effective. Working together began to feel good to both of them.

It was just getting dark when the guide suddenly stopped. He had seen signs of elephants. They got out of the Land-Rover and walked through tall brush which was over their heads. In other parts of the game reserve there was flat grassland, but here there were two lakes surrounded by high trees with vines hanging from the tops. They could clearly hear the herd coming, tromp, tromp, tromp. They watched, then ran out in front of the Land-Rover to the place in the road they thought the herd would cross. It was now sunset and, except for the birds, completely quiet. The herd started crossing. Suddenly the big bull stopped in the middle of the road. He apparently saw them and raised his ears. Then he raised his trunk and trumpeted loudly.

"Stop! Stop!" the guide exclaimed, and David realized the danger as the elephant began to move toward them. They didn't know whether to run or hide. The guide held up his wet finger to see if the wind was carrying their scent to the elephant. Then the guide put his hand up and charged the elephant, while everyone else scattered back to the Land-Rover.

The guide returned, and the bull finally wandered off; David wondered if the guide's actions had been a lot of hot air. At least, though, they had seen a herd of elephants up close.

"But I have to see a lion," David asserted. He wanted to see one for the usual reasons, but he was also thinking something else. Should he ask Elsbeth to marry him before she left for Switzerland? He had just two more days. Maya was always around, so he had no way to court Elsbeth. How could he decide? Quixotically, he told himself, *If I see a lion, this is a sign. I should ask her to marry me.*

The strange thing was, when he mentioned his wanting to see lions, Elsbeth gave him a bemused look and asked why lions were so important. "Why shouldn't I see a lion?" David responded. "All my life I've thought of Africa and lions, yet I've never seen one in Africa. I finally get on a big game reserve and naturally I want to see lions."

"But you just saw elephants," Elsbeth teased. She was now relaxed and was beginning to enjoy his attentions—a little bit. But something was happening—an odd coincidence. "Why do you need to see a lion?" she insisted again, with a touch of humor around her mouth, as if she knew his secret. And only through the oddest quirk could she have guessed.

When Elsbeth had come here two years ago, she had told herself, *If I see a lion, I will get married some day. If I don't, I won't get married.* She had ridden around the game reserve for two days and had seen hundreds of animals—but no lions. Then she had stayed at a village for two more days and finally had been driving out to go home. It had been almost dark, nearly impossible to see game. Just as she had driven around the last bend before the gate, Elsbeth had spied a lion at the edge of the road. It had stood there staring at her with strikingly beautiful eyes. Elsbeth had been stunned by its regal manner and symbolism for her. Then, it had leaped off the road.

Now, as David kept insisting he had to see a lion, she wondered, *Is he telling himself, if he sees lions then he will marry me, but if not, it will all fall through?* "Why are you so intent on lions?" she kept asking him with a merry question mark dancing in her eyes. He began to realize she knew, and it built the magic between them.

They arrived back at the hut and lighted the lanterns. David went into his room and showered. Later the women called from their room that supper was ready, and David entered to find two single beds arranged as couches with a table between them. It was already set with plates, glasses, and a big loaf of homemade bread and butter. A candle provided light. David was taken aback. He had intended for them to go to the restaurant and that he would pay. But this was precisely what Elsbeth wanted to avoid. She was not going to have him pay for her meal and play the rooster-with-the-hen role. She refused to think that perhaps she was going overboard in keeping David at a distance because she liked him too much.

It was eight o'clock and no one had eaten since noon. David suggested, "Since we haven't been going out very much, why don't we walk to the catering house and have supper up there?"

"Why should we do that?" Elsbeth demanded. "We don't have to go up there and spend a lot of money."

David didn't want to antagonize her, so he sat down. Karba sat beside him, and Elsbeth sliced the bread and served him a piece.

"Well, what's this?" he asked sheepishly when she gave him nothing else.

"What do you think it is?"

"It's bread."

"Well, what's the matter with you," Elsbeth demanded with a twinkle in her eye, "don't you like bread?"

"Oh, I just love bread. But we haven't eaten anything since noon. Why don't we go up to the restaurant to eat? We could have a real nice evening out."

"Don't Americans like bread?" Maya added, with an edge of sarcasm. She had been in the States for two years, working as a personal nurse to Helena Rubenstein, and had come away with a negative view of America. She threw in a few witty remarks about epicurean Americans, and so David had to claim his intense allegiance to the simplicity of bread. "I'm happy to have it," he insisted. "But it's worthwhile to go out and have a nice time instead of just eating bread."

"I don't see what you have against bread."

David by now had eaten several mouthfuls. "Oh. So we have bread. What will we have tomorrow?"

"Bread," Elsbeth replied, keeping a straight face.

"And tomorrow noon? What will we have then?"

"Why bread, of course."

"Can't we have something besides bread?"

"Why? Going to the restaurant costs a lot of money." They bantered back and forth, and it became more and more humorous. Finally the girls relented and suggested they go up to the restaurant. "Absolutely not!!" David exclaimed, chewing the bread with overemphasized gusto. "This is magnificent bread; why would we want anything more? Don't you girls love bread?"

Yes, they had to admit they loved bread. Actually they had canned food and meats ready to serve; by now they were all kidding each other so much they never did bring it out, but ate slice after slice of buttered bread.

After the "meal," it was bedtime for little Karba. "There's an extra bed in my room," David said. "Isn't she going to sleep in there?"

"I honestly don't think Karba would go with you," Elsbeth responded. "She's very shy. But why don't we ask her?" Then Elsbeth asked Karba in Hausa "Would you like to sleep in his bedroom in the other bed?" She nodded a yes. Then all four went to the restaurant for a Coke—Karba's first—and returned to put Karba to bed. David prayed with her and kissed and hugged her good-night.

Maya, David, and Elsbeth stepped out onto the still-warm rocks. The night glittered. David felt he could have reached out and grabbed the bright moon and thousands of stars with each hand. Brush fires in the distance, set by Africans to clear the fields, flickered bright orange in the blackness. Moonlight illuminated the bush. They looked for the Southern Cross, for David had never seen it from Jos. They finally spied it at an odd angle on the horizon.

Though they had sprayed themselves, they swatted mosquitoes constantly. There was no sound of civilization, except for the genera-

Two Weeks in the Bush

tor sounds—at half-past ten it, too, was turned off. No cars. No noises. They looked up for shooting stars and played a game of counting them. Elsbeth had a habit of always looking for shooting stars, but David and Maya were the ones to see several, whereas Elsbeth didn't.

"Look up there," David pointed. "That star is pink."

The girls looked, and Maya responded, "Oh, no, it isn't."

"It's pink. Just look at it. You're not looking at the right one." They argued back and forth, and finally Elsbeth broke in and agreed with David. "Yes, that's a pink star. It's very clear. Could it be Mars?"

David felt a flush of delight. Elsbeth had agreed with him on something!

They lay back on the warm rock and stared at the stars. David looked over at Elsbeth; he stared at her face. Did she want to be kissed? He suspected she did, but that she was shocked at herself. "I sure hope I get to see a lion tomorrow," he commented as he lay looking at the stars.

They discussed shooting stars and their origins. Maya talked about a range of subjects and around midnight announced she was going in. Elsbeth would have loved to stay longer, but she wouldn't give Maya any chance to think something was going on between her and David. She was also afraid he would come over and at least try to hold her hand. "Well, David," she observed, "that bread story was really funny. If I never see you again, I will never forget that bread story." As she said the words, she let out the tiniest gasp. David noticed and could tell her own words had shocked her, and that perhaps she didn't want the bread story to be all they ever had. He felt the same way. He didn't want to ever have to say good-bye to her.

That tiny gasp, the agreement on the pink star, the camera teamwork—perhaps she was softening . . . .

The generator and lights came on at half-past three in the morning. They had bread, hard-boiled eggs, and cold coffee. An hour later they were groggily driving out to see the animals in the dawn. They saw giraffes, elephants, and hundreds of colorful birds. By eleven o'clock they returned to escape the worst of the day's heat.

David went to lie down, while Maya and Elsbeth broke out a game. But then David came walking back in and said, "Maybe we could have some devotions." Maya was neutral about the idea, but Elsbeth promoted it. "Why don't you pick something to read?" Elsbeth asked.

David had been reading from The Living Bible in Psalms and Proverbs and was now in Lamentations. "This third chapter of Lamentations is an important passage," he announced and started turning to it. Elsbeth was taken aback but didn't say anything. How could he read "weeping songs" here? Why not a Psalm to praise nature, after all they'd seen this morning?

But David had just gone through some major conflicts in Jos. He had determined to never leave the mission field for negative reasons. Yet he was continually being squelched in a power struggle at the hospital. He'd had an inner spiritual battle over this—and had won it. Now, he was excited about this chapter's message to him.

"I am the man who has seen the afflictions that come from the rod of God's wrath. He has brought me into deepest darkness, shutting out all light. He has turned against me. Day and night . . . ."

Elsbeth watched in unbelief as David's mouth formed these sad words. It was so incongruous. She became amused. "His hand is heavy on me," David read. "He has broken my bones . . . . surrounded me with anguish and distress . . . . walled me in and I cannot escape. Though I cry and shout, he will not hear my prayers . . . . he lurks like a bear to attack me . . . . He has made me eat gravel and broken my teeth . . . ."

Elsbeth was almost laughing aloud by this time at this husky, free American in the beautiful game reserve reading: "He has rolled me in dirt. All hope is gone; my strength is turned to water." Only one line was cheerful, the last one: "There is one ray of hope: His compassion never ends."

David had thoroughly identified with the disillusioned prophet, and his heart had been thrilled by the ray of hope. The chapter's ending had given him victory in a major spiritual battle. So he was totally nonplussed as Elsbeth fell into a fit of laughter. "What's the matter?" he demanded.

"Sack of ashes! Broken teeth! After seeing those lovely animals?"

"Well," he explained, "seeing God's goodness here in the game reserve is like the ray of hope in the darkness. The verses show my need for patience for God to act."

But she couldn't be convinced. It was all too humorous. *If I were Solomon,* David thought, *I couldn't convince her.* Afterwards they prayed, then decided to eat lunch. The girls prepared a feast: *Satis* pork (like Spam), fruit salad, asparagus, beets, and cake. Now it was David's turn to be struck by the humor. He was tired and perhaps a bit punchy. "Well, now what's all this?" he demanded. He just couldn't believe they were feeding him like this after two meals of bread. The more David laughed, the more Maya stiffened her upper lip. "I don't see anything funny," she protested. Elsbeth was laughing along with David. The more David tried to control himself, the more he laughed. He was so engulfed, his stomach began hurting, and he couldn't catch his breath. He got up from the table and stepped outside. *What a way to make an impression on someone,* he thought— *laughing like a fool.* When he reentered the hut, Elsbeth deliberately repeated yesterday's punch lines, which made him laugh all over again. She was full of fun and comedy, laughing heartily along with him.

After naps they went out to the game reserve one more time. But they saw no lions. As the sun went down on the way back to the hut, Elsbeth thought, *It's a shame. I'm going home to Switzerland, Dave to Jos. I wish it were different.* It was the first time she had felt that way.

On the way back to Ngoshe Maya drove, and David sat next to Elsbeth. He felt a strong urge to put his arm around her, but at first he merely put his forearm on the seat. Then he moved his arm all the way around her shoulder and Elsbeth thought, *Oh, no!* Yet she liked it. Every once in a while he would touch her shoulder with his fingers. He hoped for some little movement, some sign of encouragement. But, nothing. In fact, she moved away from him.

Karba was sound asleep in the back seat; she looked uncomfortable. "Maya, why don't you stop for a second, and I'll bring Karba up here," David suggested. He went back, picked her up and then let her fall asleep in his arms with his sweater over her. Elsbeth looked over at them in the moonlight. Karba was so tiny. Elsbeth admitted to herself that David would make a precious father.

But David did not know she was thinking this. Elsbeth and Maya were talking in German, and he began to feel like a little boy again. They wouldn't let him drive in the dark. They made all the decisions about where to go and what to do. His little aggressions—like touching her shoulder—were rebuffed. He was frustrated. He wondered, *Is all this circumstantial? Or if I did marry her, could I be a man? Would I go around the rest of my life with my tail between my legs?* This apprehension grew when they realized they were lost and stopped at a village for directions. No one said anything about his helping. Elsbeth simply exited forcefully and strode toward a hut with a shiny, blue metal roof. David followed meekly behind with the flashlight, as dozens of Africans started assembling around them. After she talked to them, he followed her back to the car.

Froda was still awake and came out to greet them when they finally pulled into the garage. "Come over and have something to eat," she invited. They walked in and saw a beautiful loaf of homemade bread on the table. Elsbeth interceded for David—Froda made him a fried egg!

LAST CHANCE

David walked as slowly as possible with Nieck and Froda on the way to church Sunday morning. Elsbeth dawdled behind, obviously determined not to walk to church with him. She was taking pictures and assuring everyone she would come back to Africa.

David was torn between two emotions: falling in love and wanting to aggressively capture the maiden; and enraging frustrations of wondering what to do next. *She'll fly off tomorrow. I have no control over anything! Each time I score points, I end up a little tagalong anyway. How can I get her alone?*

His arrival at the church rudely shattered his hopes. Men and women were to sit separately in the cross-shaped hut. David was put near the front with the men while Elsbeth purposely sat far in the back. *He's not going to stare at me through the whole service,* she told herself. In fact, she positioned herself behind a rather large woman. During the communion service, a Nigerian was accepted as assistant pastor, and David rose to photograph him. Then David turned around and looked at Elsbeth, who returned his smile. *Ahhh, he felt, those are so hard to come by.* He went to the back of the church where he could watch her as she sang the native melodies with Christian words. He loved watching her sing, clapping her hands to the happy tunes, her head bobbing from side to side.

After the five-hour service which included farewells for Elsbeth, the congregation spilled outside and relaxed around the building, talking and laughing festively. Under a huge tree the young people were preparing to act out the story of Noah and the ark. It was celebration time, and all the townspeople were gathering; it was no small thing for an African to be ordained. There would be lots of food and music. David tried to get Elsbeth's picture in all this, but on seeing him, she'd quickly turn away. Several times he was quicker and got good shots. But he was nearly sick with frustration, standing there in the blistering heat watching Elsbeth surrounded. Once—just once —he felt a little stab of joy. He caught her aiming the camera at him—but surreptitiously, at a distance and using the telephoto lens.

He didn't see Elsbeth the rest of the day. Around eight in the evening, he felt he just had to assert himself somehow. "Froda, do you think it would be all right if I went over there?" he asked.

"Yes, I think you'd better," she responded with a smile. "They may need some help packing."

David knocked at Elsbeth's door, then unconsciously stepped back. He anticipated getting barked at, or perhaps rebuffed with a clever comment. A voice told him to come in. Maya's and Elsbeth's tone as they said "Hi" reminded him of his own reactions to a wet dog's jumping onto his lap. "How are you doing?" he asked. "May I help?"

"No, I don't think so, thanks," Elsbeth said, placing a dress in a suitcase. "Almost done."

David stood there awkwardly. Elsbeth had promised Maya she would listen to classical music with her that night after the packing. David now was an interruption to their last evening together. He stood there feeling like another suitcase in the room. But he determined, *I'm not going to get turned away this fast. It's now or never*. Finally he saw they were having trouble shutting a large box of instruments. He successfully shut it for them, and from then on he was included in the laughter and storytelling.

Maya stepped out around nine-thirty to get something, and David —determined to get Elsbeth alone—asked, "Would you go for a walk? It doesn't look as if you have much packing to do. Take a break." But Elsbeth said nothing. She simply stared at him, as if he'd just asked her to go out and catch one of those orange spiders.

She enjoyed his attentions; yet they were dark clouds over her. She had crossed romance out of her life—she didn't want to talk to him about it. She was determined to come back to Ngoshe, determined to reject romance, determined to show nothing in front of Maya. Yet here David was again.

Maya reentered the room and stayed for a half hour, then left again. Elsbeth asked David, "Well, where do you want to go?"

They walked to the hospital and made rounds on patients. Then they stood under a bright lamp outside, as if they were talking business, and David brought up his interpretations of the lions, the camera cooperation, the pink star, and the bread. He maintained she felt something for him. They stood under the light for a long time as he talked, but she gave no reply to all his observations. Finally he tried to force a response. "When we were lying on the rocks, and I had that impulse to kiss you—you had the same impulse, didn't you? You wanted to kiss me back."

Elsbeth made only a low, undecipherable sound. She would not deny it and David sensed he was right. He asked her to pray about their relationship, then walked with her rather happily on the long, dark road to her house. Though she still seemed unconvinced, as he left her off at her door he kissed his fingers and put them on her lips. "Good-night," he whispered. But Elsbeth thought, *Oh, no!* She still had no intentions of giving in to romance, even if her feelings for David were growing.

Next morning he was as frustrated as ever. He sat under a tree between the Bakkers' and Elsbeth's house. On the trip to Kano, Nieck, Froda, and Elsbeth were to ride in the battered Citroen which Nieck planned to sell in the city. David would bring up the rear in the VW, all alone. Elsbeth had given no thought to including David

Two Weeks in the Bush

in her plans; she was enthused about spending all her free time in Kano with the Bakkers. He was in the cold. Even now dozens of Africans were going in and out of her door to say good-bye. He couldn't just up and ask her to marry him—he wasn't that sure. He was even now going over the lists of pros and cons about Elsbeth. The pros had the lead by far, but . . . .

A car roared into the compound. Nieck jumped out, and within a minute Elsbeth had slipped in; they then roared back down the road. A half hour later they returned. Africans scurried about as David continued sitting with his feet up, wondering what was going on. "Lord, the ball is in Your hands," he was praying. "You got me into this. I didn't come here to fall in love. Here I am all flustered. I've done everything I can. It's up to You now. You started all this. Now what are You going to do about it?"

Nieck and Froda emerged together from the house and came up to David. They looked extremely sad. "Well, we've got some bad news," Nieck announced.

"What?"

He explained that a missionary woman had gone into labor. "We don't know if it's false labor or not. Elsbeth is really upset. It looks as if we won't be able to go with her. She's very disappointed that she won't be able to be with Froda in Kano. Looks as if you'll have to drive her to Kano by yourself. She feels pretty bad about it," he observed again, with the humor only in his eyes.

David sat under the tree, and a wry expression spread over his face and into his voice as he commented, "Oh, I don't know that I feel all that bad about this!"

Froda grinned broadly. She had been helping the romance all along and now was amused at David's impudent look. She playfully threw the glass of water she was holding directly into David's face, ice cubes and all. They laughed, and then Nieck and Froda left. *Okay, now what?* David sat there under the tree for a long time. If Elsbeth was miffed, how was he going to make progress on the trip, even if he did have her alone? "Lord, it looks as if You've done a big thing here," he prayed. "Now, don't let me mess it all up. What should I do now?"

He sat, looking at his lists, and finally decided to go see her. He knocked on the front door. No answer. He opened the door and tiptoed in, feeling he was walking on thorns. He had seen her angry before—during the symphysiotomy—and he didn't want all that fire directed at him. He didn't know what to expect.

Elsbeth was in her room alone. As she watched him approach her open door, she thought David looked like a little boy who had stolen sugar as he nervously looked around. She was fighting the events of the past few days. She recognized stirrings in herself toward David, but she was trying to reject them. As he got closer she looked at him from the semidarkness of her room and demanded forcefully, *"Why me?"* She said it not only with an edge of anger but with a deep sadness, an intense pain that evoked all the wonderful times with Claus that were now cruel memories. She had loved Claus. She saw in David the possibility of going through all that disappointment again. She felt all that pain as she demanded of David, "Why not Maya? Why not Sylvia? Why not . . . ?"

David was jolted by the ferocity of her attack. He looked at her beautiful hair and eyes in the darkened room. Her voice was harsh, assaulting. But he answered her demands with words that shocked him a bit as he heard himself saying, "Because I love you." And as he voiced the words, he felt an emotional flood of assurance and peace, knowing he was quite simply telling the truth.

There was a long, long pause after David's declaration of love. Finally Elsbeth said with deep emotion, "I don't know if I can ever love again."

She was looking at him with a hard stare that penetrated to his core. Instead of feeling crushed, he felt assured. "Well, that isn't so," he cautiously countered. "You already love. I've seen you love. I've seen your love for the people here. I've seen your love for the little children in the bush. And I've seen your love for me. It might not be very big, but it's there. Once you allow yourself to admit it, it will grow."

"How do you know I'm the one?" Elsbeth persisted. "Why not Maya? Why not Sylvia? How do you know it's me?"

Aha! David suddenly realized he had memorized his lists. "I've noticed a sense of companionship, a sense of oneness when I'm with you. I admire you. I can picture you as the mother of my children," he told her. "And yes, I could stand to look at you at six in the morning—you're very attractive. And you are a spiritual Christian." He went on and on, and then explained his reading that morning about the ideal woman described in Proverbs 31. "I could picture you in every aspect of that," he explained. "I'm sure you've been hurt, and I recognize how difficult it is. I don't want me to win and you to lose. I want you to be happy."

Elsbeth said nothing to all this. Instead, when he was finished, she stared at him awhile. Then she walked over to him as he stood in the doorway. She looked down and put her forehead on his chest. She never smiled. She simply stood there awhile, then finally suggested, "You'd better go."

David turned and walked to the door. He noticed the cook in slacks, shirt, and round African hat, working in the kitchen. The friendly old man with the mustache gave David his huge, clownish smile, and David nodded very happily to him as he left. He no longer felt like a little boy stealing sugar.

YES . . . AND NO

At precisely 4 A.M. David and Elsbeth waved good-bye to Froda and Nieck and Maya and drove the VW down the little road about 300 yards. Instead of going straight out the gate, David veered left and drove into the hospital compound. "David, where are you going?" she demanded. She sounded a little angry. "What are you doing?"

He drove around the circle and explained, "I'd like you to see the hospital for the last time." Elsbeth was silent as she stared at the buildings. David added, "You may never come back." He understood her love for the place and her hesitancy to open up to him. If they did get married, she'd have to give up so much.

He completed the circle and gave a little honk at the gate. Though it was four in the morning, the entire staff had been waiting for them and now they cheered and waved. "Good-bye, Sister. Good-bye, Sister!"

It was pitch-black with only a scrap of moon. They drove the mile and a half from the compound to the massive tree at the corner of

Ngoshe Village. He turned left and onto the deeply rutted road which zigzagged up and down creeks. He had to hit the road just right in order not to drag in the middle. He kept silence as he fought the wheel the sixteen miles to Pilka, knowing Elsbeth was having a terrible time leaving. Ngoshe had become her life and her love. She had just made the certain decision to stay and had been all excited about it and then, *Booooom!* along came David wanting to take her away. Her mind was alive with scenes like her farewell to Karba, who would go back to her stepmother. Elsbeth could still see Karba standing with one hand over her head, the other at her side, smiling at her. She was thinking of the way the Africans would cut strips of palm leaves, put stones in them, and tie them around their legs and fingers with grass; when they walked and danced it made a unique sound Elsbeth loved.

David made a sharp, left-hand turn and steered toward a gully covered by bush. Elsbeth reached over and put her hand on his knee. It was her first positive move, and it sent waves through him. He stopped the car right in the gully and leaned over and kissed her in a way that implied I love you. She said nothing, but she kissed him back the same way.

They drove on and turned onto the dirt washboard of a road to Bama. When he got the VW up around forty, they'd tend to fly over the bumps, with little traction for control or braking. The road was built up and ran through a low swamp with twenty-foot embankments on either side and no railings. Bump, bump, bump, bump. The ride was not conducive to talking.

After sixty miles they turned right and saw the blacktop highway that led to Maiduguri. Just then the sun began to rise, bright but hidden behind colored clouds. Elsbeth said, "Don't you have anything to say?"

The brightness ahead of them, and the good road, and the memory of her kiss lifted his spirits higher than he'd felt in years. "You've had a lot of roughness and darkness at Ngoshe," he observed. "But I hope that those are past—like that road we just left. I hope that your future will be like what's happening now—a smooth, straight road, with lots of light on the horizon."

They drove on a bit and finally Elsbeth asked, "Don't we have something to talk about?" David pulled over to the side of the road. "Well, yes we do." He had always pictured himself asking this question as he fidgeted on a couch, bouncing a pillow in his hands. But he had no doubts in his mind anymore. "I think we have a lot to talk about, but I guess it all depends on the first question. Will you marry me?"

"Yes," she answered simply.

They kissed again, then resumed the journey. David was delighted that Elsbeth turned into the happiest girl imaginable. The dark clouds had vanished, and she was no longer fighting against her old decision. It was as if for weeks she'd been trapped in a dark room and was suddenly let out into the light. She was like Karba dancing in pleasure. Though Elsbeth had had only an hour's sleep the night before, and little before that, she didn't want to doze. "No, no, no," she insisted when he offered. She wasn't going to miss a minute!

At ten o'clock they stopped at a restaurant in a little village and ate bacon and eggs. They really were engaged! It seemed so sudden. Everything was changed. They discussed which mission they would stay with, and their getting officially engaged in Switzerland in April, then married in August, and later taking a trip to the States. Should they marry in Nigeria? Who would come to the wedding?

They drove on to Kano and went directly to the airport. They had now been traveling over twelve hours and had to unload the crates, calabashes, and suitcases. The customs officials demanded the keys so they could search the crates. "What are you going to do with all those bags and all those calabashes?" they asked.

Fortunately, Elsbeth's knowledge of Hausa soon had them bantering back and forth with her. But they would not let her take the goatskin with the cowrie shells because of possible bugs. "What do you want an old skin for anyway?" they demanded.

"A remembrance," she replied. "They wear only this on their backs to carry the children."

"That's not true. It doesn't exist anymore," they insisted, taking the party line. "There are no naked people like that in Nigeria. Not anymore."

"What do you mean? I just worked there for three years. These are your people." But they insisted she was wrong, and she had to give the skin to David.

They were standing in the hallway, very hot, dirty, and extremely tired. Suddenly Elsbeth looked over at David and harrumphed, "*You* go to Jos. I'm not going to Jos."

David shook himself and wondered what was coming next. Elsbeth was always kidding about something. But she indignantly explained, "I want to go back to Ngoshe. I don't even want to get on the plane to Switzerland. I want to go back to Ngoshe. *You* go to Jos!" and she pushed the air with her fist, like a child shoving away spinach. The lack of sleep and multiple tensions had gotten through to her, and she suddenly believed she'd done the wrong thing. She fully saw the reality of not returning to Ngoshe, of leaving friends, of eventually ending up in Jos, and she repeated her new stance. "I want to go back to Ngoshe. I'm not going to Jos."

David tried to make light of it, but he quickly realized she was serious. He understood how tired she was and the amount of change she'd gone through. He kept silent. He drove her to the mission guesthouse and made arrangements with the woman in charge. She promptly gave David a room all the way on the other side of the compound. *Treating us like children,* David fumed. After caring for some other details while Elsbeth took a two-hour nap, he picked her up for supper. In the VW they headed downtown. Driving past a big field, they parked and decided to take a walk on the tilled ground. Elsbeth was feeling much better, and David reached out to hold her hand as they walked. Men with short hoes were building up the dirt around the dry-season corn. Others were tossing bags of dried Guinea corn onto carts.

David explained to Elsbeth why he thought she had reacted as she did at the airport. It was perfectly logical. "But if you want to reconsider," he told her, "I won't hold you to your words. You're not bound to marry me. But I know I love you. I'm absolutely sure you're the one for me, and there's no way of changing my mind. I want you to be sure of what you're doing—I know it's all happened at once. So relax. Enjoy your evening. You can go home to Switzerland and feel free. You can write me and let me know . . . ."

Elsbeth kissed him. She wouldn't have blamed him for saying, "Act

Two Weeks in the Bush

reasonable. Don't be so strange." She did relax, and they walked in the field, watching the laborers and the typical African farm scenes around them. Then they drove to the Central Hotel in Kano for dinner. It was typically British; the waiters in tuxedos had white napkins draped over their arms. Mirrors surrounded them. Colored lights shone on water flowing from classical statues. David enjoyed simply sitting there looking at her—he reached over and let his fingers intertwine with hers. After dinner they sat on a bench outside. By one o'clock, they'd been thoroughly eaten by mosquitoes and drove back to the mission compound.

Next morning, after breakfast, they stood in the long customs line as she showed her health book, passports, residence permit, and luggage. Then the plane came, and Elsbeth gave David a little kiss before walking out to the runway.

As she sat at a window seat, the events of the past few days floated in her brain like a strange dream. There David stood at the gate in an orange shirt, looking up at the plane. *Was it all true? How unexpected it all was!*

A woman sat down beside her. "You came to Kano with Dr. Christensen, didn't you?" she asked. The woman was a missionary from Jos. "He's a very nice doctor. I think he's a pilot, too."

"That's funny. He didn't tell me."

"Did you know him before?"

"No," Elsbeth replied as she looked at David standing all alone at the edge of the field, staring at her plane. "But we will get married."

4

Together

SWISS WEDDING

In the early morning on their wedding day, Saturday, August 8, 1970, David and Elsbeth walked from her home past cornfields and forest. They walked for about a mile until they came to a little hill at the edge of an ancient cemetery. The path spiraled upward around the hill, and they walked past gravestones and ancient trees. They sat on a bench overlooking the city, reading from the Bible and praying. They noticed hundreds of tombstones a few yards away. "Most of the people buried there had their wedding days, too," David observed.

"How crucial it is that we live our lives for God in our short time. Who knows how soon you or I might die?" Elsbeth responded.

They returned and ate breakfast in the small room of her parents' home that served as living room, dining room, and spare bedroom. Relatives went off to get dressed. "You're supposed to greet the people as they come," Elsbeth told him. "Someone will give you a message when I'm ready."

Elsbeth disappeared, and David realized he knew very little about this wedding. He was perfectly content to let Elsbeth handle the details; but he had been a bit jolted when told they would all take a bus ride, and after the ceremony everyone would go boating. Yesterday they had gone to a cabin in the mountains and sang, ate special cheeses, and relaxed in casual clothes with friends and relatives. What David had trouble understanding was that all fifty-four specially invited guests were *in* the wedding party. That's why there were no bridesmaids or ushers. The fifty-four people would accompany them to the church and enjoy the festivities all day with them.

David donned his suit and tie, shined his shoes, and greeted relatives. David's own parents, grandmother, and two cousins, Sherry and Carol, had come for the wedding. They had tea, coffee, and sandwiches at little tables in the backyard. Then a neighbor came up to David and told him Elsbeth was ready upstairs in her room. He wondered why the mystery. "You will find out," the woman smiled.

David entered the house and went upstairs to see his bride. He came to a door decorated with a red rose and a white ribbon with gold lettering that said Mrs. Christensen. Elsbeth was not really Mrs. Christensen yet. Technically, perhaps so. In Switzerland one must be married in a civil ceremony, and they had done that the morning before. He didn't know what this door was all about, but he knocked timidly. "May I come in?"

"Yes." Elsbeth's voice was musical and joyous.

David opened the door to a magnificent, simple surprise. The room had been decorated throughout with yellow and white flowers. Sitting perfectly posed on a little love seat was Elsbeth, her gown flowing onto the floor, surrounded by arrangements of roses. He moved close to her and gently fell to his knees to be at her height. "Elsbeth, you really are beautiful," he told her. They then kissed and prayed together. What impressed him was that all this preparation was just for the two of them. "Is anyone else coming?" he asked.

"No, this is just for us."

For ten minutes they sat and talked of the wedding and their love. It lifted their spirits. The room's beauty did not detract from Elsbeth —it was a setting for her beauty, like the green leaves around the flowers of the roses.

"Ready?" he asked her.

"Yes." They walked down the steps, David trailing behind holding her train. It was a lovely August morning. After Elsbeth had tea and pictures were taken, they boarded the wedding bus with their guests.

Historic Habkern Church is located about an hour from Berne near Interlaken. The big "mountain bus" was decorated with white carnations and ribbons. People outside would cheer and wave as they passed. David and Elsbeth sat in the back and relaxed. Everyone was talking and laughing; no one worried about finding a parking place or getting to the church on time.

They pulled up to the parsonage beside the old church, and the bride and groom greeted the pastor and entered his home for prayer. Then they emerged into a fine sprinkle of rain. "That's supposed to be a sign of God's blessings," Elsbeth said, "if you get rained on just a little—yet still have the sun."

The church bells were ringing. As they entered, David felt apprehension. He had been thankful there'd been no rehearsal. After fifteen weddings of friends, he had grown rather tired of watching brides and bridesmaids interminably practice walking the aisle in their blue jeans. But now he wasn't sure what was to happen as he walked with Elsbeth to the front of the church. The aisle was much too narrow to go two abreast; he was thankful the pews were nailed down, for he was bumping them rather vigorously. They sat down in two embroidered chairs which were decorated with flowers. An ancient organ played. As the congregation sang a German hymn, David gamely sang in German for the first time, trying to pronounce the words he saw printed before him. Elsbeth gave him a loving poke with her elbow, obviously pleased at his efforts.

The pastor preached for ten minutes (in German) on the Ninety-first Psalm. Sherry sang a song in German, then the pastor repeated his message in English. Elsbeth's brother, Wali, played the violin. Elsbeth and David exchanged vows.

During the service it had grown windy and dark, but as they emerged from the church, the sun beamed down on all the handshaking and picture taking. Then the wedding bus rumbled downhill to a hotel on the Lake of Thun, where they had coffee and pie before boarding a big tourist boat to tour the lake. David's apprehensions had long ago vanished. It was altogether the most relaxing, enjoyable day of his life. They cruised around the lake for several hours with the towering Alps above them. Sitting at a little table, they talked one-to-one with each guest as they sipped Swiss wine *sans* alcohol. Then they returned to the hotel for more pictures and dinner. During dinner one person read a poem, another a telegram, another played the piano. Finally they boarded the bus for another church where they had a family concert. Elsbeth's friends and relatives played Bach and Corelli with violin, cello, organ, and flute.

From Berne the honeymooners flew to Geneva, then Madrid, and on to Lisbon where they took a taxi to their hideaway—a white stucco cottage with red tile roof overlooking the ocean. Their cottage consisted of one big room with a curtain dividing it; there was also a little ladder leading into a loft under the A-frame.

They now had three weeks together. They sat on the beach watching ocean liners pass the drawbridge. They braved the icy ocean at midday. Elsbeth would beat David at miniature golf, and he introduced her to bowling. They ate in restaurants where they were served by formally dressed waiters.

The three weeks were joyous! One question on David's list back in Ngoshe was whether or not Elsbeth would be sexually responsive. She exceeded his hopes and turned out to be playful, provocative, and passionate.

On their last evening in Portugal they climbed into the loft with a copy of *The Little Prince*. They had been reading it aloud and had a few pages left to finish the book. David realized by now that getting into bed was the signal for talking and reading, never sleeping. He personally had not read aloud before, but to Elsbeth this meant warmth, so he turned to their place in the book and started.

The little prince was just about to be bitten by a snake and the story became sadder and sadder. David started to cry, and each word seemed to wrench more tears from him. "Stupid little book!" he complained, exasperated with himself.

"Come on, come on," Elsbeth remonstrated, hiding her grin, "Can't you even read that? What's the matter?"

David tried to go on, but he couldn't stop the tears. Then he started to feel foolish, and he began laughing and crying at the same time. Only one page was left, and Elsbeth kept egging him on to finish it. Couldn't he read a simple little book? He began laughing and crying so hard he couldn't catch his breath. He noticed Elsbeth—like a little imp—was enjoying his discomfiture. After forcing himself through to the last word, he pounced on her, and tickled her into submission.

LASSA FEVER

Panic invaded the city of Jos, Nigeria. The news was spreading fast about Dr. Christensen's illness. David was now back on staff at Evangel Hospital, but he was home with a sore throat, 104° fever, abdominal pain, and enlarged liver, spleen, and neck glands. He ached all over and could not swallow. He was very weak. Was it the dreaded Lassa Fever again? In January 1969 two nurses had died of Lassa Fever in Evangel Hospital. A year later, January 1970, another Lassa epidemic had occurred and killed more than a dozen persons. Now, January 1971, David had most of the Lassa symptoms. The timing was right for the start of a third epidemic.

He lay in bed at home, with Elsbeth caring for him. His condition steadily worsened, and soon they would have to make a difficult decision. If he did have Lassa Fever, he should immediately take serum. However, the serum was merely spun-down blood from survivors. Though it might introduce antibodies into his system to fight the fever, it could also inject new Lassa virus or cause death from kidney failure.

It had been two years ago that Lassa had first entered his life.

Nurse Laura Wine had been brought to Evangel from the village of Lassa with a strange fever. She was soon dead. Then Nurse Charlotte Shaw on the Evangel staff became sick, but no one connected the two. David and Dr. Jeanette Troup, the senior medical officer, concurred that her symptoms looked like typhoid fever and Charlotte was treated for it. But one evening David casually walked into Charlotte's hospital room and was flabbergasted to find his friend near death. She had an enlarged neck—swollen almost out to her ears. Her eyes were bloody and swollen, bulging outrageously. She panted in huge exhalations forty to fifty times per minute. A thick, gray membrane coated her throat.

David immediately called Dr. Jeanette. After a quick physical, David concluded Charlotte might have diphtheria, and Dr. Jeanette concurred over the phone. He gave her the antitoxin, plus massive doses of cortisone and antibiotics, but nothing affected her condition.

Charlotte looked at David as he worked, and he reached out to hold her hand. He was sure she was dying. "Dr. Dave, I'm going to be all right now," she gasped out. In spite of the awful suffering, she radiated a peace and faith that affirmed she was ready for death.

"Char, you're going to be all right," David agreed. He squeezed her hand. There was nothing he could do. Within moments she stopped breathing, and David sat a long time without removing her hand from his, stunned at the girl's sudden death.

Then more people died. Nurse Penny Pinneo was flown to the States for treatment, and she survived; yet a lab technician in New Jersey contracted it and died. The world was alarmed by this vicious "new" fever and the international implications.

But the epidemic waned, and by January of the next year, the time David was trying to win Elsbeth's affections in Ngoshe, it seemed a tragedy of the past. Yet he had barely seen Elsbeth off to Switzerland from Kano when a telegram informed him he must fly immediately to Jos. On arriving he was told Maiguri, his surgical assistant, had just died of Lassa Fever. David was wrenched emotionally. He had personally trained Maiguri, a thirty-five-year-old father of eight children. Ten other workers had contracted the deadly fever the past week—and one was Dr. Jeanette.

The people of Jos were terrified. Drivers would refuse to open their windows as they drove through—though it was over 100°. Foreigners were blocked from flying in. The BBC carried news of the epidemic. Evangel Hospital was largely emptied, and no Lassa serum was available.

Dr. Jeanette grew worse and worse, even though they gave her some blood from Raphael, a Lassa survivor, in hopes of her developing antibodies. At last David and two other doctors stood in her room in masks, gowns, and gloves, helplessly watching. Her neck was swollen to about twice normal size. She had gone into heart failure and kidney failure.

David walked across the room and saw Dr. Jeanette watching him. Her eyes were enormously swollen and bloodshot, bulging from their sockets, so she could not possibly have closed the lids. She was breathing in violent heaves.

David took a syringe, preparing to give more medication to her. Accidentally he broke the vial, and immediately the other doctors pulled off David's glove and inspected his hand for a puncture or scratch. Dr. Jeanette had contracted the fever from a cut during the autopsy of a Lassa victim. Fortunately David's skin was unbroken. After giving the medicine in the IV tubing, he sat down beside her and poised the needle to draw blood from her femoral vein. As the needle punctured the skin Dr. Jeanette grimaced, then abruptly she stopped breathing.

Her death made headlines around the world. If Lassa was so deadly, and there was no antidote, what if it spread from nation to nation? But before long, the second epidemic waned like the first, while researchers scrambled to find the source and develop a serum.

Together

Now, almost a year later, David knew there was no safe serum. They had sixteen units on ice at Evangel, but it was dangerous stuff. Live Lassa virus could be hiding in it. There were many ways it could kill David in his weakened condition.

About seven-thirty in the morning on the seventh day of his sickness, he called Elsbeth into the bedroom of their small, concrete-block home. He knew she was feeling depressed. She lay down beside him, and they talked about the blood tests which indicated he had a virus. But what kind? He had none of the little ulcers other Lassa victims had had in their throats—at least not yet. Timing was critical. In several cases the Lassa serum had been given too late.

David wasn't eating at all. He had to force fluids. He was jaundiced and had sharp abdominal pains. "How could I have gotten Lassa?" he reasoned in a weak voice as he stared at the ceiling. "We haven't had any Lassa patients recently."

"What about the mice?" Elsbeth observed. Saphire, the neighbor's cat, had caught many mice in their kitchen, and they had trapped fourteen in two days. Lassa hunters theorized rodents carried the virus.

"I really don't think I have it. My eyes are not swollen. The other victims had a cough and those ulcers. And it hit their systems harder." But David couldn't be at all sure. Lassa didn't affect each patient exactly the same way. He had most of the symptoms. And his was no ordinary virus.

The bottle of plasma might be an agent of life or death. They talked on and on about whether or not to give it. After Dr. Jeanette had been given Raphael's plasma, she had worsened and died just two days later. "What are the possibilities—either way?" David asked. "The worst thing that could happen is I would die. But the Apostle Paul says that's far better than living. So the worst possible would actually be a blessing for me. We shouldn't be afraid." He lay silent a moment, then said, "But I know that you would be the one to suffer."

The ugly way Lassa had killed Dr. Jeanette and Charlotte now burned in his mind. However, he had seen many people die, and it seemed to him that God gave them strength when needed. He felt peaceful as they talked about their having been married only five months and how illogical it would be for God to bring them together so miraculously and then split them apart again. Why would He have pulled Elsbeth from Ngoshe? Elsbeth was crying as they talked. They prayed for healing, for grace, and for courage. "Lord, we don't know what's happening," David prayed, "but if You want me to die, that's okay."

They decided to give David the plasma.

Next day Elsbeth sat at his bedside, the plastic bottle of Lassa serum in her hand as she adjusted the IV stand. *This plasma could kill him,* rocked in her mind again and again, but she tried to look cheerful for David's sake. He was worse today. They couldn't take a chance on not giving it. Yet what if it killed him, and he hadn't had Lassa Fever at all?

She jabbed the IV needle into his forearm and started the plasma dripping into his veins. It was pale pink, innocent looking. She trembled.

It took weeks to learn the outcome of their decision. When they finally were able to test his blood for Lassa, the lab reported no Lassa virus present. He had not needed the antibodies, although his experience proved the serum safe for others. However, it was three full weeks before his fever abated.

When he arrived in Zürich with Elsbeth for restoration, she thought he looked like an emaciated war prisoner. He was barely able to get off the plane. He had lost twenty pounds. They never learned what virus had devastated him. But to everyone's relief, a third Lassa epidemic had not hit Evangel Hospital in Jos.

Lassa epidemics did subsequently hit Guinea and Sierra Leone. It was not until June 1973 that researchers found the carrier, a small rat sometimes used by natives for food, the *Mastomys Natalensis.*

KARBA

After Switzerland, David and Elsbeth extended their health leave to America—the last nation Elsbeth had wanted to visit. But she found her former attitude was mostly based on stereotypes gained from books and magazines. "I thought all America was like New York," she observed after arriving. "Now I even think differently

Together

about New York!" She found the tollgate police courteous and even many New York subway riders rather friendly. She and David drove to Chicago and got snowed into a motel. Both found that their bodies had so adjusted to Nigeria's heat that they could hardly tolerate bitterly cold weather.

When they returned to Nigeria, David was anxious to get to work. Immediately he was pressed into an extremely busy schedule. Evangel's outpatient load alone was seven thousand per month. One day he stepped briskly into an examining room where an unmarried missionary woman sat waiting. After greeting her, David asked where she worked. "In the North," she replied.

"Where?"

"Way up near Maiduguri."

"Which village?"

"Oh, just a little village way out in the bush." Nigeria has tens of thousands of villages.

"I've been up near Maiduguri. Which village do you work at?" David insisted.

"Barawa."

"Oh, do you know Karba?"

The woman's face lighted in excitement. Of the sixty million people in Nigeria, he would know little Karba? Fourteen hours away? But suddenly the woman's face turned sad. "Well, Karba, she's a pretty poor kid. The other children stoned her a few days ago. The chief's children go to school, but she had to stay home to take care of the goats and the sheep. The older she gets, the more she's becoming a slave."

David and Elsbeth, who was now eight-months pregnant, had been praying for Karba a great deal. David knew Elsbeth thought about Karba often, and that evening he brought it up as they sat in their yard. Multicolored butterflies flitted by, tropical birds screeched and flew amid flowers, trees, motorcycles, noisy old autos, roosters, and guinea fowl. As he related the conversation about Karba, Elsbeth couldn't keep herself from crying. She knew that Chief Musa tried to be good to Karba, but he couldn't protect her all the time.

They went in for dinner. Previously David and Elsbeth had talked of bringing Karba to Jos for schooling. Africans often give children to relatives for several years, and they wondered if Musa, who liked Elsbeth very much, would give permission. Previously, Elsbeth had pushed the idea away—she didn't want to use Karba or spoil her. But after this report . . . .

Elsbeth soon delivered a boy, Erik, by Caesarean section. Six weeks later she and David, along with her visiting parents and "Nana," David's grandmother, drove a Land-Rover to Barawa. As they pulled up to the huts on Thursday afternoon, Elsbeth saw Karba in the distance; she was naked and carrying a head pan of manure. The little girl hurried to her compound to put it away, then came running to them. Elsbeth hugged and kissed her, despite flies and filth. Karba had a high fever, was coughing, and her belly was still distended from malnutrition. They found that Musa was at another village trading cows, so they asked permission to take Karba for a few days.

At Ngoshe they treated her and had her sleep on a cot. On Monday Musa's brothers arrived for a morning visit, and David invited them in for breakfast. The Nigerians had never eaten cereal, so when David broke out the Corn Flakes, they munched them enthusiastically while the whites explained their idea about Karba. Musa was still gone, and David tried to be very diplomatic. "Think about it. Take your time. If you say yes, we'll arrange for Karba's transportation to Jos."

On Tuesday morning it was time to say good-bye to Karba again. It was always painful for Elsbeth. Karba wore a school dress with a little scarf. Her coughing had subsided. Elsbeth hugged and kissed the six-year-old. "Now, after school," she instructed, "go right back to Barawa. Good-bye now." She waved to the little walking figure. It was already hot when Karba left for school—95°—and the round trip was sixteen miles.

An hour later, much to David and Elsbeth's surprise, Musa came walking along with Karba. His brothers had sent him a message, and he had intercepted the little girl along the path. He fully approved of their taking Karba immediately. "Karba, do you really want to come?" Elsbeth asked her. The little girl beamed back her approval. "It's far from here," Elsbeth explained. But Karba was overjoyed, and Musa saw them off with a great display of friendship.

But the trip which followed turned out to be rather traumatic for a little girl who had scarcely been beyond the huts of Barawa. They drove the 150 miles to the airstrip at Mubi where a plane lands about once every six months. To the villagers, a plane was an *event!* David and Elsbeth found the red-and-white plane, an Aztec with six seats, surrounded by black waves of people in robes, turbans, and colorful leg bands. About five hundred Nigerians were massed on the grassy strip. As they were about to board, a man started directing the people to back away. Few would move, so he started to push very roughly and to threaten with his whip. His yelling and shoving increased the chaos, but soon all the Africans were off the runway. All except one—Karba. She was standing next to Elsbeth; the man, thinking she was a disobedient child, yelled at her, rapped her on the arm, and grabbed her forcefully. Then he literally threw her into the crowd.

Elsbeth ran! "No!" she screamed as she plunged into the mass of people and grabbed the trembling child back. "She belongs to us!" "Well," the man with the whip gruffed, "I didn't know."

As the five adults took off, Erik in Elsbeth's lap and Karba in David's, the little black girl was still shaking visibly. Not only had the man's roughness frightened her, but she had never even seen a plane before, let alone been inside of one. During the entire two-hour trip, their explanations couldn't abate her fear. She sat with her eyes staring straight ahead, absolutely refusing to look down. She finally put her head on David's lap. Only as they came down on the runway in Jos did Elsbeth get her to look out. "See, Karba, this is just like in a car. Look at the homes over there!" Then they drove to the city, and Karba stared at the new world alertly, but silently.

They wondered if Karba were intelligent enough to do well in school. They put her in second grade, and within a few weeks she proved more than capable. She went from the bottom of the class of thirty-five to the top. By June, although she spoke only Hausa, Karba was one of the family. Since Erik was only six weeks old when Karba joined them, he looked on her as his sister.

Eventually David became Karba's legal guardian. That fall, he took her to Switzerland; Elsbeth had gone ahead weeks before with Erik. When they arrived at the snowy, windblown Zürich airport, Elsbeth greeted them and was jolted by the new Karba. She looked positively European, wearing tights, a windjacket, hat, and gloves. "There are towers of Babel all over the place!" Karba remarked in fluent English, awed by the airport. "Where is Erik? Why didn't you bring Erik?"

She missed her little brother, but five days later she had two brothers. Boris was born in November 1972. Berne was blanketed in snow, and Karba got to stay high up in the Alps and attend an old-fashioned school. The little black girl romped in the deep white stuff, sang Swiss German songs and experienced a Swiss Christmas.

5

Train to Serikin Pawa

"Let me come with you!"

Elsbeth loved mothering Karba, Erik, and baby Boris. But she yearned for two things also—David, and the bush people of Africa. With David's extremely long hours at the hospital, she enjoyed little time with him. And she deeply missed Ngoshe. David was to visit the dispensary in Serikin Pawa, deep in the bush. He was immediately enthused about her joining him.

They arrived at the train station at nine in the morning with Don-Lami, David's Nigerian dispensary supervisor. David walked into a storeroom. People were sprawled on the floor, a boy was urinating, and a man sitting at the desk was utterly dwarfed by piles and piles of paper. David purchased the tickets. Printed prominently was the statement that a passenger could not hold the railroad responsible for anything that might happen to him. At two o'clock the train's arrival was announced by a loud playing of the national anthem. By four o'clock they were finally on their way in a stifling-hot caboose which was jammed with people, live chickens, pots, pans, goats, and sacked corn and peanuts. Elsbeth grinned at her husband jammed in beside her. European trains were never like this!

After a half hour they stopped by some huts; villagers rushed toward the train, screaming and jumping on, while others tried to sell rice, sugarcane, and fish. Some tried to sneak on without paying; finally amid great commotion, the guard waved a red flag, and the train started off again.

At a larger village David and Elsbeth got off to eat. The scene was beautiful. Huts on the right were framed by tall palm trees, banks of trees were on their left, and the train arched into the horizon as it stretched around a bend. In the distance they could hear the cadenced sound of men carrying heavy loads.

Their grunts grew louder. *Uuuh! Uuuh! Uuuh!* Elsbeth had watched Africans make their loud, grunting noises as they pushed heavy furniture on carts. As the sounds grew closer and louder, they realized the grunts must be coming from many men. Then they saw them in the distance, not walking, but quick-stepping single file, each with an enormous container of milk on his head that must have weighed two hundred pounds. *Uuuh! Uuuh! Uuuh!* The men grunted loudly in unison as they filed past David and Elsbeth, scores of Fulani nomads in delicate balance—sweaty black torsos thick with muscles. On and on they filed past as David and Elsbeth continued eating. Then the men unloaded their precious milk. Suddenly, shouting and commotion erupted in the front. Elsbeth wondered if the train would jerk and take off any second. Children around them screamed, babies urinated, and everyone jostled for another quarter-inch of space. A long time passed. Finally the Fulani men groaned and swore as they filed back to unload all those containers of milk. It was the wrong train! One by one the men now grunted past them with their enormous loads on their heads. *Uuuh! Uuuh! Uuuh!*

A watchman came and lighted the kerosene lanterns. They started off. *Choo-choo. Clackety-clack.* They peered at the passing villages in the twilight. On and on they rode, until at last they arrived in Serikin Pawa at eleven that night.

David and Elsbeth pried themselves out of their cramped positions. Then they walked through the markets. They followed a path for a full half hour; huts and trees were lighted by a half-moon. *"Bature. Bature."* ("White man.") They heard the shout racing all across the village as they walked. Children whispered as they walked by, *"Bature! Bature!"* Then church members came running to greet them.

David loved watching Elsbeth as she talked with the Africans. She knew their idiom well. Both felt so at home here, so relaxed. But their one-hour train ride had already stretched to fourteen hours. David inspected the dispensary, and they had to return.

Back at the station David tried to buy tickets, but the ticket agent was "off seat." It was two in the morning. Lanterns hung on trees and posts. Groups of Africans talked, sang, and danced. The smells of hot food, goats, chickens, cows, horses, motorcycles, and human perspiration blended surrealistically with the night sounds. Singing. Gambling. Drumming. Selling. It was a carnival! Don-Lami brought mats, and they lay on their stomachs, jammed together in the crowd. Elsbeth's hand sought out David's, and they smiled at each other nose-to-nose. David felt a sudden sensation of joy at her closeness, her sexually provocative wink, her love of being here with him and "her people." They dozed.

Phweet! At four in the morning a sharp whistle blew, and they snapped upright. The passenger train was coming! It chugged up to the station, and David saw that all were freight cars except for three packed passenger cars. The full surge of humanity around the train elbowed, shoved, and muscled into the cars. Someone called and helped to pull David and Elsbeth into the car. They tried to sit on some bags but were so jammed they couldn't move. The car was already stuffed at several times capacity, and beyond all that was the *kaya* ("goods").

The shelves above the aisle and the space between the seats were jammed with *kaya*. Colorful baskets and bulging bags of onions, beans, and Guinea corn rose higher than the seat backs. Chickens squawked loudly. Not only other people's chickens, but now David and Elsbeth's chickens! They had been handed to them as a going-away gift. Finally David glared at his noisy possessions and shouted, "Squawk! Squawk!" back into their faces as they scratched and insolently pecked at him. Though Elsbeth and David couldn't see each other, they laughed as if they'd been dumped into a wacky movie.

Away the train went with all windows open and, before long, stopped at a village. People immediately threw *kaya* out the windows and jumped after it. As David and Elsbeth tried to find space on the floor with the onion and bean bags, they found themselves once more rocking back and forth. They tried to sleep; but each time they dozed, the chaos of village stops would jolt them awake. Both were exhausted from the heat, lack of sleep, and the stench, but were strangely enjoying their experience. It was especially funny when the conductor, wearing standard uniform and hat, came along checking tickets and used the only means possible for getting from one end of the car to the other—he balanced precariously as he walked on top of the seat backs.

David decided sleep was impossible. He asked Elsbeth for a banana and reached over like a contortionist for it. He was sitting on a bag of onions, and the strong odor mixed with the banana smell as he peeled it. But he took a bite. Then, a huge roach landed right on the end of the banana. He looked at the roach. David's hands were filthy. He didn't want to touch the banana. Elsbeth saw the little drama and started laughing. David finally decided the roach couldn't be any dirtier than he was, so he blew it off and finished eating his banana.

A Yoruba man, who was hanging out of the door, was dismayed when his tied-up chickens broke loose. There was much squawking and fluttering and stirred-up dust. A man in front of them ripped meat from bones with his teeth and spit out the gristle. After swallowing his meal, he reached down for a paper scrap from the floor and started working the chunks of meat out from between his teeth. To their right, a Yoruba woman roughly elbowed a sleeping Hausa girl when her head would drop on the woman's shoulder. Others on the train exchanged glances disapproving of her rudeness. Most of the people were extremely warm, immediately exchanging smiles. They seemed like instant friends.

David was cramped and decided to stand awhile. Suddenly they heard a strange, fluctuating Arabic singing. *"Ahhhh. Aaahhhh."* Two blind men, one big and the other small, were inching their way through the car. Passengers warned them there was no space, but they persisted, singing all the way, eyes rolling unconnectedly. Both were dirty and greasy, but the singing was very good. *"Ahhhh. Aaahhhh."* The big man had huge teeth and opened his mouth so widely David could see right down into his throat from the other end of the coach. They felt their way along the seat backs, almost stepping on a sleeping man's head. He warily woke up and joined the others in exclaiming, "Go back! Go back! No room!" *"Aaahhh. Aaaaahhhhh."* On they came, singing and moving closer and closer to David and Elsbeth. Once in a while, someone would hand the beggars a coin. They never broke stride as they precariously balanced on the jerking, swaying train, singing all the way. Then they hit an impasse. The *kaya* and people were so packed at one point, they could not go one inch farther—and that point was right next to David, who was already pinioned by the *kaya*. But both men rammed themselves in beside him. *"Aaaahhhh. Aaaaaaahh,"* they sang loudly in his ear. Yet David felt like putting his arms around them. He respected these men who were doing their best, trying to survive, bursting out in song despite their blindness.

"There is such a need for dispensaries like the one at Serikin Pawa," Elsbeth observed as they rode. "But they need so *much* help! Wouldn't it be wonderful if we could live several months in each village? You could do the surgery and teach the dispensers, and I could set up the clinics."

David did not need to think a long time to feel enthusiasm for the idea. At Serikin Pawa they'd felt like a team. He had worked with her previously on obstetric cases and considered her a colleague with exceptional judgment. He felt a strong pride in her love for the Africans and her ability to work with them. And with a plan like that they could have more time to be together. They could be partners and fulfill her deep longings for both motherhood and meeting the awesome needs of Africa's people.

"If I could choose anywhere in the entire world to live," she explained, "I'd pick a little village like Serikin Pawa. I just love the people. They're so easy to relate to. Life is uncomplicated. A slow pace—but we could slow down, come down to their level. And maybe it's not down at all. Maybe it's up. Their life is so simple, like our going back to the farm. So you have to carry water for a mile. So what?"

They talked on about their dream. But for the immediate future, other demands were forced on them . . . .

6

An American Autumn

LABOR DAY

It was early Saturday morning, September 1, in the Pocono Mountains of Eastern Pennsylvania. David and Elsbeth, with their three children, had come to the States for a year's furlough and further training. Elsbeth sat in the small living room of David's Aunt Esther's house, looking at a big maple tree which was just starting to turn color. *What a lovely setting,* she thought, looking at the splotches of yellow and red on Mount Minsi. *Why do I have to feel so lousy when I finally get a vacation?* She had hardly slept the night before. She felt nauseous and weak and couldn't eat. On checking, David had heard a loud heart murmur, and he had ordered blood tests. Her hemoglobin was shockingly low. Was it chronic malaria? Another tropical disease?

David ate breakfast and then helped her into the car. He drove carefully on the potholed dirt road, then through the steep hills of Delaware Water Gap. Elsbeth looked at a clump of golden trees which were so shrouded with fog that the leaves were dripping. Then they were on Route 80 and in five minutes turned off at the little reflector sign marked Hospital. *We've passed that sign before, while going to the shopping center,* she mused, *and I thought, wouldn't it be nice for David to work in a little hospital here in the Poconos?*

David had to help her up the front steps. As soon as they opened the door, they heard the blare of loudspeakers paging staff members; there were aides wheeling patients and accident victims talking. It was becoming a bloody holiday weekend in the tourist mecca.

"Can you wait a minute?" the harried receptionist asked. Staff members were running. Patients sat in wheelchairs. A boy with a broken leg winced in pain.

"No," David answered. "We at least need a chair." Elsbeth was trying to stand, but then fainted.

They put her on a cart and wheeled her to a small examining room, where they had her put on a hospital gown. A sixty-year-old woman lay groaning on the other bed, her husband sitting beside her. David and Elsbeth looked and both knew immediately that she had terminal cancer. She let out a cry of agony, and her husband tried to comfort her, saying, "The doctor will be here soon."

A doctor finally walked in. "Well, Mrs. K., are you back? We'll give you four pints of blood, and that should relieve the symptoms. Then you can go home. That's all we can do for you." Elsbeth looked at David and locked onto his eyes. *Boy,* she thought, *a few words and that's it—into a coffin. How she must be suffering!*

The hematologist entered the room. After drawing some blood from Elsbeth, he asked about the malaria smears and the various tests she'd just had. "How did it start?" he asked kindly.

"With a headache." Elsbeth told him of the shortness of breath as she climbed stairs, her weakness, and nausea. To Elsbeth the doctor looked a little nervous. He couldn't tell how her past malaria was affecting the tests. "Well, I'd like to do a bone-marrow test," he announced.

As soon as the doctor left, Elsbeth exploded. "Dave, they are really crazy! Here we come from the tropics. I could have hookworms, any kind of worms. But they have to think the worst!" Elsbeth's miffed feelings showed in the tightness of her mouth as she lay under the green towel. A bone marrow test was unpleasant. Deep down she felt the edge of fear.

"Look," David responded, touching her face, "we've got to do it. You could have cancer or something."

They wheeled Elsbeth to another room. A boy was lying on the other bed, and they drew a curtain between them. The hematologist held in his hand what looked like knitting needles. He asked her to face the wall and gave her a pain shot in the left hip. "Mrs. Christensen," he insisted, "you can be sure that today of all days—Labor

Day weekend—I wouldn't be doing this if it weren't important. We're up to here with work and a short staff. You have to trust me."

They went in with the needles, which did not create much pain. But as they sucked in the marrow, the awful pressure almost made Elsbeth cry out. They returned Elsbeth to her room, and she lay there, glad it was over. "Listen," David said, "I have to get a bite to eat. I'm starting to feel weak." He left, and Elsbeth looked over at the cancer patient. The blood from the bottle hanging beside her was dripping into her arm. She was groaning less now.

What do I have? Elsbeth kept asking herself. *A minor virus? A blood anomaly? Cancer?*

She waited. And waited.

Suddenly words came blaring over the loudspeaker. "Dr. Christensen. Dr. Christensen." The officious tone roared like an icy arctic wave, smashing into her, drenching her. Why would the doctor want to see Dave alone?

She lay there, full of dread, sweating as she tried to pray. Was the news really going to be that terrible? The door stood open into the dark hall, and as she stared into it, Elsbeth could see something in the distance, coming out of the darkness toward her. All she could make out were the bones of David's face coming closer, his eyes sunk far back, like smoldering coals.

"Dave, is it bad?"

"Yes, it's very bad." He sat beside her and took her hand.

"What do I have?"

"Leukemia."

She breathed out and let her arms down on the bed. "Well, which kind?"

"The worst."

"Uhhh," she groaned, and her whole body trembled. Yet she felt weirdly as if the whole thing were happening to someone else.

David had seen the slides of her bone marrow. "It's acute leukemia. Unless there's a miracle," he said soberly, "you will die."

They wept. Eventually the hematologist entered and talked to David about going to Temple University Hospital where they had facilities and expertise. It was also close to Havertown where they were planning to live for the next year. The doctor left, and Elsbeth got up very shakily to get dressed. The older woman getting the blood looked over at her as they were finally ready to leave.

"Bye-bye," the husband said from her bedside. "Good luck."

David and Elsbeth walked out of the hospital still crying. She felt as if she were weeping like a child who'd lost a favorite doll, but she couldn't turn off the tears. The sun was illumining the colorful trees and green bushes. The early afternoon brightness irritated Elsbeth. *If only it were dark,* she thought, *like what's happening to me.*

David drove back on Route 80, back through the village, back up the gravel hill and pulled in beside the big sun porch. Karba stood there looking at them drive up, and Elsbeth started to cry again. Karba's face broke into weeping too, and she asked, "Mommy, are you very sick?"

"Yes, I am very sick."

David's parents and aunt and uncle questioned Elsbeth. "I have leukemia," she blurted out, crying and returning the embraces. "I must go to Temple right away and I may not live."

Everyone was soon weeping. Elsbeth and David packed numbly. Finally they dropped the suitcases into the trunk. Elsbeth held Erik and Boris close, kissing them and Karba and thinking, *I may never see them again. In fact, I probably never will see them again.* Elsbeth looked into their faces and kept promising them, "*Daddy* will be back. *Daddy* will be back."

It was late afternoon and a bit misty as their wheels lifted dust on the dirt road. They drove slowly, silently. Elsbeth had not gotten to see much of America, or the Poconos. As they passed trees and little lakes and the Delaware River, they all whispered to her to stay, to enjoy, to see more of the beautiful countryside.

They stopped at a Howard Johnson's for a cheeseburger and cola, and then continued slowly down Route 611. Arriving in Philadelphia they turned on Broad Street and saw in the dusk the great gray shapes of the Temple medical buildings. They turned left at a stoplight and parked in front of the emergency ward.

Elsbeth had never been to Philadelphia before, and she didn't know that this was the sort of neighborhood people were afraid to come to, even during the day. It was hot and dirty as they walked up the steps. Black policemen. Black patients. Black staff members. She felt as if she'd walked back into Africa. *Like home in Ngoshe,* she thought, warmed by their blackness. A boy sat with a badly gashed head. Several men lay drunk. A man with a broken leg turned painfully on a stretcher. Children were screaming.

A nurse escorted them to the sixth floor and a nice room overlooking the lights of Broad Street. In the distance was Independence Hall with its Liberty Bell. A nurse took her blood pressure, then put a tag on her wrist. *Like I'm marked in prison,* Elsbeth thought. The nurse put her to bed and then took her temperature—it was 101°.

An intern who had been alerted that this was an emergency asked questions, and David gave the history. "Doctor, may I have some aspirin?" Elsbeth asked. "I have a terrible headache."

"No, we have to wait. Aspirin might affect the blood." Immediately the intern started sticking her for blood samples. Tubes and tubes and tubes. The intern was a kind, friendly man who would sit down and talk and show concern. But he was new and not adept at drawing blood. Elsbeth had good veins but he would try eight to ten times before success and would "blow" the veins, spreading blood into the tissue. Other doctors came and asked all the same questions. She was still refused aspirin, and she felt like wringing the necks of the doctors every time they told her no. Would it really make *that* much difference in the samples?

Another doctor came in, and three or four doctors examined her all over again and asked the same old questions. A resident asked if anyone had done a malaria smear. More tubes and blood. In and out, in and out. Nurses. Interns. Residents. Her fever was mixing her headache into a soupy, foggy pain. Elsbeth felt she was going crazy.

David watched the intern's shaky hand jab at her veins. Elsbeth winced in pain. "Oops, I'm sorry," he would say, and at first David rode with it, knowing interns have to learn, somehow. He had learned years ago. But watching her veins get blown one by one built his helpless anger. They weren't just dealing with fevers, charts, samples, books. They were treating a person—Elsbeth! He tried to be understanding and spoke softly; but he wanted to protect her—to protect her veins—for they'd be her life-support system if she had leukemia. As the process continued hour after hour, he started to feel like tearing the interns apart. Yet if he sounded like a crank, he knew they'd both be treated like cranks. Finally, around one in the morning, he expostulated to the intern in as cool a way as he could. "Look, please lay off her. It's time to let her sleep. She's had a bone-marrow test. She has a splitting headache. These needles are like bees—poking, probing. She has to keep retelling her story. Give her an aspirin and sleeping pill. Let her alone!"

The intern assured him they would. Elsbeth glanced at Dave and thought he looked like a ghost. "You'd better go home, Dave," she told him.

He nodded and kissed her, then left.

But they didn't lay off. More tubes and tests. Elsbeth felt she was on the edge. She was weeping. "Listen," she declared indignantly, "I will run out of here if you don't get away."

They tried to soothe her and she fell into a more pensive mood. "I want to see my children," Elsbeth said.

"How old are your children?" the nurse asked.

She told about Boris, Erik, and Karba.

"Oh, you'll see your children again. Don't be so dark," the nurse cautioned. But Elsbeth saw in their faces the belief she was dying.

They poked and examined her till dawn, taking many tubes of blood—which "required" over fifty assaults on her veins. She had cried and cried and cried. Finally they gave her blood, and almost immediately she felt better, as if she were suddenly a different person. By eight in the morning her headache was gone, she no longer felt dizzy, she could even walk around. As her mind began to clear, she prayed, "Lord, I want to go home. This can't be happening to *me!* It's a nightmare. I'm ready to wake up now!"

She lay back on the bed and looked at the tube carrying blood to her veins. It was finished, the vein was blown. Blood was oozing. She rang the bell. No one came. She rang it again, then a third time. She had not slept all night and felt everyone had forgotten her. She began sobbing—Elsbeth couldn't stand being trapped in this room. The morning light and the trees outside tantalized her with their colorful life.

Then someone was standing in the doorway, an old man with a

little mustache. "What's the matter?" the man asked kindly. "You look upset. What's wrong with you?"

"Yes, I'm upset!" she nearly screamed at him. "I just came back from Africa and I have leukemia. My children are still in the Poconos, and my husband went to Havertown. We just found out about it, and I just can't believe it. I cannot stand all this . . . ."

He stood there in the doorway listening to her, nodding at each detail, but beaming out peace. "Well, whatever it is," he told her, "even if the diagnosis is right, put yourself completely in God's hands." And to Elsbeth he strangely looked—in his gray-haired graciousness—like God Himself watching her. He came to her bedside and read the Twenty-third Psalm aloud. Then they prayed together, and Elsbeth thanked the dear old pastor from a central Philadelphia church who was up early on a Sunday morning to visit the sick. She felt a degree of peace, and a conviction that God had specifically sent His messenger to her.

David woke in the morning feeling hot, dreary, and doomed. He had been in this home just once before, with Elsbeth, and they had been excited about bringing their family here. Now he rose, ate, then walked through it alone and out to the car. He thought back a few years to the vultures he had seen circling over the Nigerian troops. The winged doomsayers seemed to be in his own sky now, following his car effortlessly. Great squadrons of them seemed to circle the hospital as he parked his car.

When Elsbeth told him the doctors hadn't stopped their diagnostic work till five in the morning, he was furious. Her story of the old pastor who had just left eased his emotions a bit, but both still felt as if they'd been dropped out of a plane over a hostile country and now were in the hands of the torturers. No one meant ill; the white-garbed workers meant it for good. But their actions often hit David and Elsbeth as cold, at times unnecessary, even brutal.

They sat dazed. David remembered that when his sister, Lois, had died, people had given tidbits of advice and things to read. But even the Bible had been hard to focus on back then; all he could do was see through blurred tears. It was the same now. He dabbled at a Gospel of John, the same one he had tried to read the night before as Elsbeth was being probed and jabbed. But it was no use.

Someone brought Elsbeth lunch. David walked downstairs for his, then returned and sat by her again. They talked of sin and illness and where pain and suffering came from. It was numbing, sitting there hour after hour.

The blood gave Elsbeth strength, so they took a walk. Within the huge complex was a little chapel; they entered and sat on a pew near the back. David pulled out a hymnbook and tried to read, but he couldn't. They tried to pray but ended up weeping again, their heads against the backs of the pews.

They cried and prayed for an hour. How were they to pray? For healing? God had allowed the illness. They prayed for the children and how they would face this, and Elsbeth thought, *It's like praying at my own funeral.*

They rode the elevator back to the sixth floor. Visiting hours were almost over. "Before I go, let's read the Bible," David said. A verse had come to his mind as he had showered that morning: "I am the resurrection and the life. He that believeth in Me, though he were dead, Yet shall he live! Yet shall he live!" He located the reference in the Gospel of John in The New International Version and started to read chapter 11 aloud. He paused after he read verse 3: "So the sisters sent word to Jesus, 'Lord, the one you love is sick.'"

The words exploded in David's mind, so strongly he almost gasped. *The one Jesus loves is sick!* It wasn't just the person he, David, loved. Elsbeth was the one *Jesus* loved. He had trouble continuing his reading, and both of them cried again. Then David read, "When he heard this, Jesus said, 'This sickness will not end in death. No, it is for God's glory . . . .'"

David and Elsbeth each had a Gospel of John in hand. The fresh, new translation was shocking—it had never stood out like this, and they literally read the last phrase aloud ten times, wondering if this really were for them, and if so, what it meant. Was the Lord saying Elsbeth's sickness wasn't unto death? They didn't know. If God had allowed it, should they cringe from it, trying to escape?

They read on through the chapter, for the first time in their lives fully sympathizing with the bereaved Mary and Martha. They sensed God's higher plans as Jesus stated, "I am the resurrection and the life. He who believes in me will live, even though he dies; and whoever lives and believes in me will never die. Do you believe this?"

And then they read those simple words that couldn't be improved over the King James Version:

"Jesus wept."

Here we have been weeping all day, David thought. He remembered a friend on the phone that morning saying, "Disease and death are from Satan. Our world's topsy-turvy. God weeps with you and He hates sin and its results. He hates disease. He sorrows with us." David felt that Jesus hadn't grown two-thousand-years worth of calluses on His emotions. He cared just as much for Elsbeth. Jesus had shouted, "Lazarus, come out!" This same weeping God asserted His power and raised him from the dead. Lazarus's cells were all messed up, his platelets, red cells, and marrow were disintegrating after four days of decay.

If God could do that for Lazarus, why not Elsbeth's bone marrow?

God could reach down. God was in control. And as they reread the chapter, they cried again, but this time it was not hopelessly or out of self-pity. In this darkest day of their lives, they had been like children in a pit, and God had reached down and thrust them into light and love. They felt as if they'd been thrashing in water all day and now felt a rock under their feet.

DIAGNOSIS

Dr. Joseph, an energetic Jewish woman in her forties, remembered David from his student days here at this hospital. She took full charge of Elsbeth's case.

"Be honest with me," Elsbeth asked firmly.

"I want to see the slides first," the doctor replied. "I don't want to believe the worst yet."

Elsbeth lay in the quiet room, waiting for her to return. In about a half hour, she walked back in and sat down in a chair. "You can ask whatever questions you'd like," the older woman offered.

"I would appreciate one thing. If I have just one week to live, or a month, or whatever, I want to know about it."

Dr. Joseph nodded. "If you don't get treated, you have from one to three months. With treatment you have a fifty percent chance for a remission. If you go into remission, you have eight to eighteen months before a probable relapse."

Elsbeth tried to interpret the numbers into life and kids and days with David. "What if I have only five months? If I have to be in the hospital three of them, I'd rather just go home and get blood and what I need to relieve the pain."

"No! You have good chances!" The doctor exuded hope for her, and Elsbeth could feel in her expressions almost a cheerleader's desire that her patient plunge into the battle, plunge in to fight toward victory, no matter what the odds.

More tests were run during the rest of the week, and Elsbeth was allowed to go home Friday for a brief time. There was a slight chance—very slight—that a drug Elsbeth had been taking since Boris's birth had produced the dreaded symptoms. She had a bad rash over her stomach and down her legs. Her lungs and heart were normal. When she had enough blood, she felt fine. All the data was to be presented to the top hematologist. Another sample of bone marrow was to be analyzed.

At home David and Elsbeth prayed, hardly daring to hope that perhaps it wouldn't be leukemia after all. It would be like a fairy tale materializing before them if they were told, "Go home. It's all a mistake. She'll get well!"

They waited in high anticipation on Tuesday in Dr. Joseph's office for her to come back and deliver the news. Would the Lord do the miracle they had prayed for? But as Dr. Joseph entered the room, Elsbeth saw dejection in her face.

"Is the marrow any better at all?" Elsbeth asked.

"No, it is worse." she answered.

Elsbeth felt as if someone had taken a rough-edged brick and smashed it into her face. As they walked out of the hospital to the parking lot, she tried to understand. *It seems every time in my life when I am totally happy, I get stopped cold.* She thought of the day when, as a seventh-grader, she'd gotten a new pair of shoes. She had been so proud of them, with their little buttons on the side! She had put them on for the great feast in Berne—the day they closed down the trams, and people could throw confetti on the police and celebrate with the crowds. But a woman in the shoving and pushing had accidentally stepped on one shoe, tearing it, ripping off a button, and Elsbeth had felt as ruined as the shoe.

She thought, too, of the time she had said to David one night in Africa, "Dave, I'm almost afraid it can't last. Our marriage is almost too complete. We have it so good."

She got into the car, and they started out of downtown Philadelphia toward the suburbs. Less than a year ago she had been sitting in her parents' home in Berne at the Christmas season. She had just given birth to Boris in a tough C-section delivery. There she had sat at her childhood home with three healthy children. Snow had blown outside. Her parents had set the table for a little snack. Christmas music had been playing. Erik had chattered away. The perfect, newborn babe had been lying quietly. Elsbeth had physically felt chills as she exulted in the perfect moment; yet at the same time she had thought, *If something as wonderful as this is so close, is not the opposite around the corner?*

They passed block after block of skinny homes which looked like suburban homes sawed in half, then glued together fifty at a time. Black children in loose, flying clothes ran in front of them. Next block, the houses were the same, but the children were white. What different scenes she had seen in her life! What varied emotions! She thought of the wonderful days in the forest with Claus, then his incredible phone call, and the killing of her genuine, powerful love. *I've become a pessimist,* she thought. *I don't want to get hurt. When I emerge like a snail out of its house, then boom! I get hit. Is the Lord trying to teach me not to look on earth as all good? That earth isn't my home? Do I love this life too much? So many lessons. But, oh, they get rougher and rougher.*

If Elsbeth thought moving back into Temple would be like entering a morgue, her roommate dispelled that instantly. She splashed her own color and laughter into their little room. She was a small Jewish lady with a cute, upturned nose, blonde hair piled high on her head, square blue-tinted glasses, and a warm hug for everybody. Her long-haired husband pumped David's hand vigorously as they met. He had the same verve as his wife. Mr. and Mrs. Fineman exuded a warmth that took them by surprise.

"Mind if I call you Elsbeth?" he asked after supper on the day both women were admitted. "We can't call you Mrs. Christensen."

"Sure. That will be fine."

"Now, Honey," he said to his wife. "What could I bring you?"

"Apple pie and Coke. And please bring Elsbeth something."

"No—that's all right," Elsbeth demurred.

"Oh, come on, sure you want something," he insisted.

"Actually, I just had supper. I think. . . ."

"Whaat!! the wife insisted. "Do you like apple pie?"

"Sure."

"Do you like Coke?"

"Sure."

Elsbeth was grinning with them, and ten minutes later Mr. Fineman was back with apple pie and Coke for everyone. They laughed and joked and watched TV and ate pie. Then he asked her, "Elsbeth, do you mind if we ask you why you are in here. You sure don't look sick. My wife has been passing out frequently and we don't know why. Suddenly she just falls. The doctor says he needs to do tests on her."

Elsbeth had hinted a little at her own diagnosis, trying to avoid the cloud it would bring. "Well, I have leukemia. I came in for chemotherapy."

"What do you mean?"

"Yes. I have leukemia."

Suddenly they were shocked out of their humor. "Well, that just can't be," Mrs. Fineman insisted. "They must be wrong. You have rosy cheeks and you look so healthy."

They talked on about Elsbeth, and as she showed them pictures of Erik and Boris and Karba she started to cry. They choked up with her. "Elsbeth, I just believe," he said, "that if you have leukemia, you'll get well again. We're not religious Jews, but when it comes to this point, we will pray for you. God will do it! It just can't be."

Then they cheered up, and Elsbeth couldn't help but be swept up along with their good humor. After her husband left, Mrs. Fineman put her hair up in curls, wrapped a scarf over them, and sat in her long robe on top of the bed like a reigning queen. She discovered the red buttons which raised, lowered, and tilted the bed, so she promptly took command of her ship. Elsbeth thought she looked like a fisherman in a boat (complete with fly hat) as she went up, forward, back. Both of them began laughing till the tears were coming and their throats were almost hoarse. For a half hour she played commodore of her little vessel—forward, backward, up, and down. And Elsbeth, who had dreaded so much coming back here, thanked the Lord for her buoyant roommate.

The Finemans continued their natural therapy. He would bring *TV Guides*, newspapers, chocolate cake, pie, soda. He kept offering to take David to dinner at Fisher's, an expensive restaurant nearby. Mrs. Fineman was always on the phone in between her tests. She would return from the tests in a wheelchair with a triumphant, "Well, another free ride!" When the announcement came over the loudspeaker, "Visiting hours are over," Mr. Fineman would lie on her bed snoring loudly, even though the instructions were repeated five times. Mrs. Fineman watched a late movie one night and explained it to Elsbeth, since the volume was set for just one person. The awkwardness of explaining the plot became another cause for laughter.

That week Elsbeth could still take walks around the hospital with David. Her white-cell count was high enough so that she wasn't in danger. But then she developed a hangnail. Soon her whole finger was throbbing. By Sunday evening she had a fever and had to be transferred to a private room.

Chemotherapy is a frightening gamble. White cells—both cancerous and healthy—are wiped out, leaving no leukocytes to fight invading germs. A simple cold could now kill her.

Elsbeth's fever rose to 104°. She had contracted septicemia, and her body was defenseless. The doctors tried to fight the infection with antibiotics, but without effect. She was given copious amounts of blood and platelets. The IV needles were permanent fixtures in her arms, one for infusions, the other running to keep the vein open. She was also in complete isolation—anyone entering her room had to wear a gown, mask, and gloves.

Elsbeth grew so weak she could not lift her arm; the pain was excruciating. David would help her all day and until ten at night. Then, after going home, he'd answer telephone calls. Often staff blunders heightened the discomfort. IV's would have to be restarted unnecessarily. Nurses would barge into the room at three in the morning and turn on the lights—without apology. The loudspeaker paging doctors was on at full volume in her room all night. Both David and Elsbeth felt they were trapped, unable to fight the system, with Elsbeth too weak to cope. She knew she was very close to death.

On the fifth day—her birthday, September 22—the antibiotics started winning the battle against the fever. She felt a little better and eventually got up, took a bath, and cared for her flowers. As she got a little stronger, she wrote some letters and stared out at the cloudless weather with its colorful autumn trees lining Broad Street. She had not been home to Switzerland in the fall season for seven years, and she had very much looked forward to the smells and crisp air of autumn. Now she was trapped behind windows, with normal life moving briskly outside them.

One day Mrs. Fineman, now discharged, walked in with her husband who held three huge boxes in his arms. Winter coats for Karba, Erik, and Boris! David and Elsbeth were amazed at their thoughtfulness. And in addition to Dr. Joseph, many of the staff showed compassion and concern. Especially Angelo. He was a Catholic medical student from a little village in the Poconos. He and Elsbeth talked about missions and communicating Christ while ministering to people's physical needs. He was a tonic to her. About four in the afternoon one day, she heard running footsteps and scuffling of feet in the hall, then Angelo's voice saying, "No, no, it can't be! This must be the wrong room!"

"Well, it's 618," another voice insisted.

Angelo sounded apprehensive yet dogmatic. "No, it can't be!" Then he threw open the door demanding, "Here, let me check."

Elsbeth looked up at him from her sitting position on the bed, book in hand. Angelo's normally rosy cheeks were white, and as soon as he saw her he exclaimed, "Oh, thank Jesus!" Behind him stood two medical students with a cart, whom he turned to and talked with for a moment.

"What happened?" she asked Angelo.

"You will understand," he said sheepishly. "I saw them, from down the hall, coming to your door. I knew it was your room, and they were here to take a body to the morgue. But it was the lady next door who died. Elsbeth, I knew it couldn't be you. Not so fast as that!"

But when David came later and Elsbeth told him the story, she said to her husband, "Let's face it. It could have been true. It could have been me."

At the end of three weeks, Elsbeth was getting more and more deeply depressed. More chemotherapy ahead. A good chance she would never go into remission. Was anything but pain and hospital walls and death ahead? "Dave, I just don't know if I can stand any more," she said flatly.

A few minutes later Dr. Joseph barged into her room with slides in her hand announcing, "Take your mask off! Take off the gown! You don't need it any more." She animatedly showed David the bone-marrow slides. "It's like it's from a different patient," she told them. "The cells are coming back! You'll still need another treatment, but you can go home for a few days."

Elsbeth was packed in fifteen minutes. "Dave, let's not waste time calling," she suggested, walking hurriedly from the room. It was now the end of September, and patients and staff had known her so long that one after another showed surprise as they walked down the hall. "What? You can go home? Wonderful!"

The freedom of riding in the car in the clear autumn air, after the gown and mask procedures, was exhilarating. Yet Elsbeth was apprehensive. She knew how quickly little children forget. Would they really remember her—remember her as *Mommy,* not just another of the women caring for them? She asked David that question six times before they pulled into the driveway.

They sneaked in and saw Karba in the living room. The girl's face became almost a physical scream of delight, but Karba somehow swallowed the sound as Elsbeth motioned to her for silence. Then Erika, a Swiss girl friend of Elsbeth's who was now tired and beat after weeks of caring for the kids, saw her friend from the bedroom. She had no such ability at silence. She let out a loud scream, and the two young women hugged each other. Boris pulled the bottle out of his mouth and looked up at Elsbeth and giggled. Then he giggled some more in a very distinct recognition as Elsbeth reached out to hug him.

Erika pointed to the bathroom and Elsbeth tiptoed in. Erik was sitting in a little, yellow plastic tub, scrubbing away, his back to the door. She watched him for a moment. Then he saw her, and his mouth opened in a gasp as he exclaimed, "Hi-ya, Mommy!"

She picked him up and hugged his wet body against her. She felt her children had been given back to her again. David stood in the doorway weeping.

After a week at home, Elsbeth developed another fever. Her white blood-cell count was still low. Once again she would have to battle infection through antibiotics.

This time she was assigned to a different room. As they walked in and she looked around, she grew increasingly upset. "Dave, I can't even see the sky from this room! You know this is where they bring unconscious patients before they die. Not even a tree—just a parking lot. This room is horrid! Ugly. I just *can't* stay here!"

David tried to calm her down. "Get undressed and I'll come back," he promised.

Before long he was walking in with three vases of beautiful fall flowers to liven up the room. Elsbeth stared at them and let their beauty crowd out the ugliness of their new setting.

But the ugliness of the diagnosis couldn't be so easily dispelled. She was soon getting injections every four hours. Then a new bone-marrow test showed she wasn't making red cells. Elsbeth knew she couldn't live without them. It wasn't typical, and Dr. Joseph couldn't figure it out. She was worried. Elsbeth began praying about the red cells and asking others to join with her.

One couple, the Shephards, wrote, "We are praying very specifically that you will make red cells and that the Lord will touch you." The morning it arrived, Elsbeth held the letter in her hand and reread it, praying that God would answer all these prayers and touch her that day.

A brief time later she heard Dr. Joseph's short, marching steps coming down the hall. She could always tell her walk—feminine, determined, assured—but this time her pace was much faster than usual. Dr. Joseph had not waited for the elevator, and she now snapped into the ugly room breathless from her run up the stairs. She wore no gown and mask but a bright red dress under her white smock. "I have to sit down since I am absolutely out of breath," she exclaimed, "but I have to tell you that your marrow is *loaded* with red cells. You're in remission! You can go home!

7

Lausanne

HOME IN BERNE

Elsbeth sat in the flowered yard of her parents' home on the outskirts of Berne. It was July. She'd lived with leukemia for ten months. Her remission had held; though she experienced pain, uncertainty, and treatments in America, she had enjoyed the snow, and the spring flowers, and trees in her backyard, and her children kicking a ball at the fence David had built. She'd seen Karba adjust in school, wowing her classmates by carrying in an entire tray of milk cartons on her head each day. She had entertained, and visited Longwood Gardens, and reveled in the hibiscus, orchids, and great palms.

Now, in Switzerland, the sunset framed an old house and tower in the distance to the west of the grammar school she had attended. In front of her stretched a wide field of wheat, and beyond that was an inviting pine forest and the mountains she had lived with most of her life. She had careened down the little hill below on a sled.

Erik and Boris were charming Elsbeth's relatives. Karba was fast picking up German. They all loved watching the horses coming down the streets and visiting a farm with pigs, chickens, and goats. They were also happy victims of jet lag. Normally up at six in the morning, Erik could be still sleeping soundly at nine when Elsbeth would peek in at him, and Boris would barely be moving before noon. David slept in with them and would waken with swollen eyes. Yet the boys took their naps and went to bed at their regular times, which gave Elsbeth extra time with her parents and brothers.

She felt as if she had tumbled back into her childhood: the same home, yard, and forest—even the same fish pond she had splashed in as a girl. She kept telling David how wonderful it was to be here.

The church bells were ringing. It was precisely eight in the evening. Elsbeth could hear the much fainter cowbells after the church bells died away. At night she would awaken to hear gentle tinkling as the cows munched their grass in the big field.

If only gentle cowbells typified her dreams. Instead, her subconscious whirled with a sense of doom. One night she had dreamed:

> She was on a ship. A man was stamping on the hands of black men and women who were hanging—out over the water—from the railings. "Stop that! They will die!" Elsbeth exclaimed, but he kept doing it. Then someone said to her, "Watch out. He wants to kill you, because you shouted at him." Elsbeth then looked out the window, and there he was, pointing a gun right at her. She panicked, but then the police took him away. She relaxed for a moment—but then, there he was again! The police had let him go, and he was aiming the gun directly at her, about to kill her . . . .

Elsbeth had awakened so terrified she had literally been unable to speak. She realized the symbolism of cancer and the man with the gun, of remissions, and then death back at the door.

At times she felt bitter: *I'm dying, and God isn't doing anything to stop it. Who is going to be the mother to my children?*

Here in Switzerland she enjoyed the good Swiss bread, the yogurt, and fruit. She talked with her parents and brothers and played with her children. She was enjoying each individual day. But the man with the gun was still at the window.

THE CONGRESS

Elsbeth and David rode two hours on a train from Berne to Lausanne. Then they boarded a bus crowded with delegates to Lausanne 74, the International Congress on Evangelism. It was a lively scene, with some people in native costumes and some in business suits. Elsbeth was surprised at the handshaking and talking—a Swiss bus was usually quiet. Here were strangers from a dozen countries, already talking like old friends.

The bright flags of the nations flapped at the entrance of the huge exhibition hall. Everything was superbly organized, with young men and women in Swiss garb waiting to help the delegates. They pinned on tags which included their names and languages, for example, I SPEAK FRENCH AND ITALIAN or I SPEAK JAPANESE. Delegates in colorful African robes, Indian saris, and even an American Indian with feathered attire mingled in the lobby. Many stopped and read where David and Elsbeth were from and then shook hands. Camaraderie flowed as they talked to Brazilians, Indonesians, Britishers, Canadians and Pakistanis. Over four thousand Christian leaders had come to participate.

David and Elsbeth sat near the back for the first meeting. Each delegate had his own set of earphones which he could switch to any language. Massive TV screens magnified the speakers so that everyone could see each gesture and nuance.

They found themselves sitting behind Mrs. Billy Graham and her daughter. As Graham began preaching, David saw him with Ruth's slightly graying hair and face framed in front of his. *What a temptation it would be,* David thought, *to pull on his sleeve at this Congress and say, "Billy, this is my wife, Elsbeth, and she has leukemia. Would you pray with me for her healing?"* If anyone could evoke His power, couldn't this man of God? But they had determined: No! Here also were four thousand mature Christian leaders. If anyone would know something of faith, prayer, and healing, they would. But David and Elsbeth had given their lives to evangelism and they came as part of that continuum. They had already gone to a Kathryn Kuhlman meeting. They had no intuitive knowledge that God would heal her, and they waited for God's leadership.

In some ways they felt as if they were in a perpetual desert. During the last years in Nigeria, David had been extremely busy. Now the leukemia had stretched their spiritual resources. The Congress started a kind of healing. Like many others present there, David was particularly impressed by the concern and urgency. It did not seem sentimental nor contrived—it flowed through the delegates.

They walked into a meeting of the National Strategy Group for Nigeria. When the Nigerians saw Elsbeth walk in, they stood up and cheered. Many of them knew she had leukemia. David and Elsbeth recognized about thirty people who had been patients or co-workers. They watched Stan Mooneyham of World Vision show giant slides of Africans dancing in pagan rites, then report on God's dramatic working in their lives; the spotlight then turned to the man on stage who was at the center of what God was doing in Africa. Mooneyham repeated the procedure for Brazil. He illustrated again and again that God was alive—He was at work—all through the world!

David joined a session on the Holy Spirit. One man gave his reasons for speaking in tongues and everyone, including opponents, applauded him. David was deeply impressed that these delegates could disagree but still show a maturity and concern for each other.

David also attended a buzz session on evangelism and the arts. The leader loosened everyone up by putting the participants into a big circle and relating stories and illustrations. Then he separated people into groups, and David joined one of about twenty persons. A German commented that the problem was the Americans were running things, but an Australian reacted, "My brother, if it hadn't been for the Americans, we wouldn't have this Congress." Again, their spirit was not vindictive. *That ye may be one in the Spirit* flowed through David's mind. *We're individuals. We debate, but we have one Spirit.*

Each group in the buzz session then had three minutes to illustrate a concept. They were given three words: *Love, Hallelujah,* and *Mercy.* David watched one group send out a man who pretended he was stricken and fell down crippled. Another man came walking along, then stopped, and stooped to pick him up. The three joined him. Soon everyone was raising the helpless man up, and as he rose he started to unfold like a flower. After he had been lifted high above their heads, the once-stricken man opened his arms to the Lord and shouted, "Hallelujah!" Everyone in the room clapped and cheered.

As David was being caught up in the spirit of this Congress, he thought back to the only other time he had ever felt quite this way. He had been singing in the New Jersey All-State Chorus in Atlantic City. Everyone had memorized the music, and they responded as one to every little move of the conductor. Singing that day, David had hardly known his body had existed—he was part of that one organism singing in concert. And here he felt the same—like one, a unit of a body genuinely dealing with the world and its problems.

While David was in the buzz group, Elsbeth had taken a bus to a tea for the ladies. She arrived at one of the big hotels at the lake and got into a receiving line. "Could you save me a place?" she asked Erika, who had come with her. Erika nodded, and she quickly ducked out to a phone to call the lab for results of her blood test.

The news was ominous.

She reentered the receiving line, her spirits chilled. She shook hands with Ruth Graham and Leighton Ford's wife. She stood around with the others, drinking tea in the ornate dining room. She then sat down in a chair in a back corner. A Japanese girl sang a solo. Billy Graham's mother said something. But Elsbeth was thinking, *Seventeen blasts—cancer cells—a very bad sign.*

Elsbeth was silently weeping as Ruth Graham spoke, but she tried to concentrate. The evangelist's wife was saying that sometimes God asks us to do very hard things—things we don't want to do. There was a time in Ruth's life, in China, when she had to say goodbye to her parents and go to school. She did not want to leave her parents and prayed half the night that God would let her die. Yet God did not answer that prayer in the way she had asked.

Ruth then related how people ask her, "Aren't there times you're lonely, with your husband gone so much?" She admitted that, yes, she had problems. But there came a time when she realized Billy had problems, too. "When he comes home, do I cheer him up, or add to his burdens?" Ruth realized she shouldn't run to her husband with every little problem. There was a person she should run to first—Jesus. Then, when her husband came home, she would have the inner strength to help him with his burdens.

Elsbeth thought of David. *If I first put this before the Lord, He will help me. And when I have to tell Dave about these blasts, I will try to cheer him up.*

Her intentions were brave, but she could not stop the flow of tears. Tomorrow there would be a bone marrow test; the next day—what . . . ?

THREE MEN

David was on the phone again. He was having trouble getting through for the latest medical report. It was Wednesday, the last full day of the Congress. This morning he and Elsbeth had run eight blocks to catch a train—and she had beat him! She seemed in wonderful condition.

But what would the lab report be?

The doctor came on the phone. Yes, she had 21.5 blasts. The red count had dropped. "But don't get excited," he told David. "Go through with your vacation plans." But David saw it as a confirmation of the inevitable. He scheduled another test for Friday and hung up the phone.

He was melancholy as he walked through the crowds seated at tables for lunch. He saw a small round one on an upper balcony which had an empty place. The three men seated there greeted him warmly as he sat down. They passed him the Swiss casserole of noodles and cheese. He spooned some out and took some salad, but he wasn't very hungry.

The man on his right was a Nigerian with an unusual spiritual dynamic. The other two were Australians.

"Don't you feel well?" one of the Australians asked.

"I'm fine."

David wanted to avoid talking to anyone, but the men kept probing, "Well, my wife isn't well," he finally admitted.

"Oh. Well, what's wrong with her? Is it serious?"

"Yes."

David was forced to explain she had leukemia, and right away the response was, "Well, have you prayed about it, brother?"

It seemed an almost insulting question, though sincerely meant. "Yes, I have prayed about it."

"Well, then, can't you claim her cure?"

David swallowed and watched as a waitress poured a cup of coffee at the next table. He chewed on some bread. "No, I can't claim her cure, because I don't know whether the Lord wants to cure her. Obviously He doesn't. We have been praying, and here it is coming back."

"Maybe this report is a good thing," the Australian offered.

"No, I am sure this is *not* a good thing."

David halfheartedly spooned his pudding into his mouth as the men asserted that David's problem was a lack of faith—that he

Lausanne

wasn't claiming the cure. David argued vigorously against this view: "Yes, I can pray in faith. But the answer belongs to God. I can't tell God what to do. I can let Him know what I want Him to do and what my heart wants. I am praying for her healing—but I have to leave the answer to Him. I can't claim what I don't know."

They argued back and forth for almost an hour. One of the Australians was dark-skinned. He looked David directly in the eye. "Weren't you at the Crusade Sunday?" he asked kindly.

"Yes."

"Was your wife there?"

"Yes."

"I saw you outside the service and told myself, *There is a man who needs prayer and has a heavy burden on his heart.*" David felt his observation was probably not unusual. He had brought Elsbeth from Berne in the train Sunday. She had vomited all the way down and vomited outside all during the service. He had not been cheerful.

The Australian also told him that the three of them had gotten together every night to pray, "Lord, lead us to someone with a need." And now David had sat at the one empty place at their table.

The other Australian was black-haired, but with a lighter, olive complexion, a bit chubby, and considerably more vocal. It was he who was most aggressive in arguing with David, and the Nigerian had been siding with him.

"How can you say you don't know?" the lighter-skinned Australian asked. "Hasn't God given you anything?"

"Yes, He has given me a verse. But I haven't known how to interpret it. I don't want to take it out of context."

"Well, what is it?"

"It's the verse we read the Sunday we learned of Elsbeth's leukemia. 'This sickness is not unto death.'"

At that all three men tensed up in their chairs. "There you have it! God has given you the answer." Now, even the dark-skinned Australian was siding with the other two. Surely here was a message from God. Why not just claim it?

David had often thought about just that. Had he been negligent? Was he bringing needless grief to himself? Or had that verse been for that specific Sunday—for the *remission?* "God is sovereign,"

David insisted. "His thoughts are beyond mine. Even if He allows evil, in the end it's for my good and Elsbeth's good, even though our hearts are crying in pain. I can't see that God is allowing this because of a lack of faith on my part—faith is hearing what God has to say and acting upon it. I don't know what He has to say regarding Elsbeth."

Perhaps he was arguing too much. There was the coincidence of their prayers and his coming to their table. He was certainly ready to pray with anyone, and these men were obviously sincere and concerned.

They left the table and entered a little room as another group was gathering. The men put four chairs into a circle, then each man prayed specifically for Elsbeth's healing. Each repeated a verse that came to mind. They prayed that God would reverse the lab report, that it wasn't evidence of a recurrence, that God would completely cure her now.

Don't let me be a doubter, David prayed silently as he listened to the others. *If this is what You want to do—do it, Lord. Don't let my doubt affect the prayers of these men.*

As David prayed, this verse came to his mind: "Call unto me, and I will answer thee, and show thee great and mighty things, which thou knowest not." She shared it with them, and they were thrilled. They shook hands and departed, asking David to let them know what happened.

By this time David was late for the next session. Instead of going to it, he walked down a few flights of stairs to a tier overlooking the population clock in the center of the lobby. As always, groups of people were standing around contemplating the millions of babies being born. Slide pictures of children were displayed next to the clock. The stairs from the lobby rose to balconies and classrooms above. David turned and stepped into a pavilion shaped like a wigwam. Slides on creation and life were playing constantly, flashing from a carousel. It was a good place to be alone.

For an hour, he prayed. "She's in Your hands, Lord. I'm in Your hands. You're in charge. We want her healed. We also want what You want." David asked for peace, but also realism. He felt ecstasy for a fleeting moment, but no rising convictions of healing nor floods

Lausanne

of joy. Nor could he condemn himself for having a heavy heart. All he could say was, "You know, Lord."

He rose and walked to the Francis Schaeffer buzz session. The theologian was sitting at the front of a room in a relaxed manner, with his Swiss boots on the desk. He wore knickers and a white turtleneck sweater. David strained to catch the lip movements above the gray goatee as he answered questions, for the microphones were not working. About a hundred people were grouped casually around him.

The mikes began working. Schaeffer responded at length to numerous questions, then gave time for just one more. Hands went up. Someone started talking, but Schaeffer interrupted. "No, no, I saw that fellow back there, in the pink shirt, with his hand up."

So David rose and asked, "How should we interpret so many verses like, 'If you ask anything in my name, believing, it shall be done for you'? If God doesn't answer in a favorable way, is this because of lack of faith? People say, 'Just claim healing. Claim it! God says it, so claim it!' In a sense that's what happens in salvation. Whoever calls upon the name of the Lord will be saved. The Bible says it. I call—therefore, I'm saved. It's as simple as that—taking God at His Word. So the same argument goes for healing. God says, 'You have not because you ask not.' Okay, I'm asking, and God said it. Therefore she's healed—but she really isn't. Now what do you do with that?"

Schaeffer answered that God does respond directly to our prayers and that He is not trying to manipulate us. But in all of Schaeffer's explanations, four of his words echoed with a ring of truth in David's mind:

Let God be God.

David found himself repeating the phrase, "Let God be God."

After the session, an Indian man maneuvered through the press of people and came up to David. He was short, brown, and wearing a brown Nehru jacket. He shook David's hand as he said, "Brother, I want to thank you for asking that question. It is very meaningful, especially to me." For the next ten minutes, he spoke with conviction and love about seeing various missionaries claim healing for persons who later died. One missionary claimed the healing of his wife and everyone claimed it with him—yet she died. "However," the Indian said, "that same man got a tremendous victory. I'll never forget that father walking along behind the casket, with his two children—one in each hand—with complete peace and obviously accepting God's will. His showing God's peace in the face of death had more impact on his community than if God had healed her." He went on to explain that he had been praying for the healing of his own wife for years, but God had not seen fit to restore her.

LAST DAY IN SWITZERLAND

David and Elsbeth rushed to arrive early for the communion service. Everyone expected a moderate turnout, but they were amazed to see almost everyone there. After his message, Billy Graham asked for a fresh dedication to serve Christ in the world. Elsbeth wondered as she stood with the other delegates, *How can I serve the Lord? I was willing to serve in Africa. I am willing to go back. But God, who is almighty, wants me to serve Him with leukemia. I feel willing to accept Africa, but not leukemia. Yet I must. This is my new mission field. This is how I must serve Him.*

Her tears were flowing. She reached for David's hand. It was almost noon. She knew in five minutes he would have to call the hematologist for the final report. She sensed it would be bad. Each report was like someone was sharpening a knife—sharper, a little sharper, each time sharper. Yet she also felt the Holy Spirit in almost a physical voice saying to her, "Don't give up. Just trust. This, too, has passed before God's throne. He could have stopped it—but He let it pass." And she felt His peace inside. It didn't matter if she were to die. It mattered what she did for eternity. The whole concept, though old to her, grew fresh and vibrant.

She gripped David's hand. This rededication as they stood here was like another wedding vow. It was one thing to stand in front of the altar, happy, ready to take new steps together. It was quite another to vow near the end, knowing they were both in God's hands. Elsbeth heard Graham comment as he said farewell that this precise group would never meet again on earth, but they would surely get together in heaven.

David went to a phone and after a time elbowed back to her

Lausanne

through the assortment of delegates. He held her in the hall as people rushed here and there for planes, kissing, yelling good-byes, waving, shouting. He was subdued. "Yes, it really looks like a relapse."

Instead of going directly home, they decided to take a train ride into the mountains. They entered a train with enclosed seats on one side only. The entire right side was glass. Light rain misted the magnificent mountains and lakes as they sped along. An Italian family sat in their booth, and David was amused that, although Elsbeth usually insisted she couldn't speak Italian, she was chatting away with the family.

Eventually the sun broke through and they could see the mountains and lakes more clearly. As they passed the Lake of Geneva, Elsbeth pointed out the beautiful Chateau de Chillon jutting out over the water. "A Christian named Bonivard was imprisoned there, tied to a stake for four years or so," she told him. "When you go in to visit, you can see the path he wore into the stone floor by his pacing. It must have been terrible in winter—an open window with bars, no protection . . . ."

David watched the castle as the train moved by it. His arm was around Elsbeth, and he drew her closer to him. "God has a job for each of us," he mused aloud. "What if you were that man? Someone always seems to have it worse."

They changed to another train to go up into the mountains. They began going through long tunnels and found themselves jumping up and down to shut the windows because of the awful noise from the suction. Yet they also enjoyed the moments of solitude, sitting in silence, unwinding . . . .

They stopped in a little village. A young doctor dressed in his whites was saying good-bye to his girl friend. She got on their train. David was seeing Switzerland in the rough, off the tourist trails. Some stations were full of geraniums, others barren. They saw the dark brown huts where the Swiss poor eked out their hard life, where children went on skis to school. They stared at rocky, angled peaks, wide valleys, little chalets . . . . Elsbeth talked to David of the rustic cabins one could rent. She had wanted to hike here with David, as her brother and his wife had done. "Funny," she said to him as she looked at the mountains, "how it depends on where you are when you read the Bible. What does 'white as snow' mean to a Nigerian? And to the Dutch, what does 'I will lift my eyes to the mountains' mean? But to the Swiss!" *Switzerland is so little,* she thought, *but it has so much—the lakes and mountains, the countryside, the rough villages where people struggle for their little wheat.*

Suddenly Elsbeth realized that this would be their last train ride together in Switzerland. She started crying. Why couldn't she have another nice week here as they had planned? "It reminds me of children's water colors," she told David. "There's so much that's wonderful here. You put the colors on to make a design, and the colors blend together. The black moves into the other colors, and you don't want it there, but it mixes in, making all the bright colors dark."

They did not even get to stay the weekend. Friday noon they learned she had 70 percent blasts and a low white count. David didn't wait for the bone marrow results but booked the next flight out. They left the children with their grandparents amidst tears.

They made it back to Philadelphia just in time. Her white count had zoomed from 5,000 to 200,000 in one week. The swelling and rapid multiplication of cells made her bones like pressure cookers. By Tuesday, the pain was intense as Elsbeth lay in her new hospital bed.

Yet her perspective had changed. Her task focused into that room. She and David had a job to do that no other person at Lausanne could do. God was at work all over the world. This hospital was their mission field. God had His plan—even though they might never fully decipher it here on earth.

They could trust Him.

8

A Weekend in August

FRIDAY EVENING

"What a different person you are without pain," Elsbeth said, her hair half covering the pillow on the hospital bed. "Pain is a terror, like something creeping inside. Especially when it gets to the lungs. Even with the shots, when the pain comes, I can't breathe deeply."

David sat beside her. "Is that the worst part?"

She held up her hands about a foot apart. "If this is normal breathing, then this"—she held a thumb and finger one inch apart—"is how much I can breathe. It's like a throbbing finger coming up from the waist, and as it rises it cuts off my breath." She paused. "Yes, in one way it is the worst. I was always terrified to be under water or trapped in smoke where I couldn't breathe."

A few days before, when Elsbeth was in agony, a doctor had mentioned *fibrosis,* and the word slashed into David's emotions. He remembered from medical school the fibrotic process where the bone marrow becomes full of scar tissue. Was this causing the pain? Would this be permanent? Yet Elsbeth's pains would change location. Were they from reactions to drugs? Dead cells thrown into living tissues?

"Right now it feels as if I have tetanus," Elsbeth explained, opening her mouth and gingerly moving her jaw. "Stiff. I feel stiff all over."

When she had come in on Monday, she had been feeling fine. Now, twelve days later, she had endured long seiges of pain, IV's, blood samples, nausea, good days, and bad days. The decision to come to Lankenau Hospital had been a great relief to Elsbeth. Temple was the scene of all the terrors of the last seige, and the cheerful surroundings of the room, with trees and grass visible outside, made it a new experience instead of a return to an old nightmare.

A lab technician walked in with a tray. She stuck Elsbeth in the forearm, and David watched Elsbeth's eyes as they stared at the blood slowly moving into the long, thick tube. *What's in that blood, that deep-red stuff like living wine? What new cells? What cells gone wild?*

The tube filled slowly and Elsbeth's eyes stayed on it. David knew there was almost no chance at this moment that the blood test would show anything, but how could their doctor be inactive in the face of death? It was like the old man he'd just left who was dying of emphysema. He'd given him a Vitamin B-12 shot, only because the man had requested it.

The technician left and Elsbeth held cotton against the puncture site. Her platelets were extremely low, so her blood would barely clot. "Last night I suddenly felt wet," she told David. "I was bleeding from the hip puncture."

Voices in the hall suddenly flowed around the corner and into the room. Two of David's cousins and a girl entered cautiously. Introductions were made.

"How are you doing, Elsbeth?"

"Pretty well, thank you."

One cousin pointed to an autumn poster (with the bright reds and blues of mountains, trees, and a large lake) covering the entire wall next to her bed.

"That's really nice. Come with the room?"

"No," Elsbeth replied. "It belonged to Lois. Dave brought it from his office to brighten the room. We don't know where the lake is, but a girl in here yesterday said she's sure it's Maine."

"You have beautiful flowers, too," he said, walking up to bright red geraniums and a white lily on a shelf opposite her head. "But they're not real." Elsbeth laughed. "They don't allow real flowers here. It's so strange. At Temple I was in complete isolation. Everyone coming through the door would have to wear a gown, gloves, and mask. But it was a joke in a way, because you couldn't keep everything sterile. I remember a young doctor coming in with all this getup, having gone through the sterile procedure, and he started to hand me a packet from Switzerland. Then he caught himself. 'What am I doing?' he laughed to himself. 'Here this packet has been all over Switzerland picking up germs, and here I am handing it to you.' Yet at Temple I could have flowers—lots of flowers and plants. It was a virtual garden."

The conversation soon turned to the greeting cards taped in neat rows on the walls and standing on the dresser. "So many precious people," Elsbeth told them. "I can't wait to get home and have the whole bunch over!"

SATURDAY

For breakfast, David ate his usual bite-size Shredded Wheat with raisins and drank a cup of Sanka. Because Elsbeth asked him to, he gave some milk in addition to regular dog food to Prince, their Swiss mountain dog. *Dumb, alongside of a German Shepherd,* he thought as he tossed him parts of a doughnut Elsbeth had sent from her tray for Prince. *He misses it, even if I practically hit his nose. A German Shepherd wouldn't. But he's obedient. Friendly. Good with the children.*

Water the plants. Check the mail. Close the windows. He'd grown to depend on Elsbeth, and now he felt a bit like a scatterbrain as he grabbed his doctor's bag and got into his white Plymouth with the sticking doors, leaking window, and fresh bird splats on the windshield. He had started a private practice, which was time-consuming. He was frustrated by all the little chores undone—the wide red-and-gray bricks he'd carefully placed in the spring now sinking into the mud. *How ordinary life is, even with leukemia,* he thought as he drove. *But you can't escape that hospital room. Any second she could call, needing me. It's like being shoved into a giant wad of bubble gum. You try to walk away, and it all sticks to you.*

He stopped in to see Elsbeth, then went to the Saunder's House nearby where he had numerous elderly patients. *When I'm old, I'll want someone to care about me,* he thought as he listened to complaints about ringing ears and blurred vision and other symptoms of disintegrating bodies. In one older woman he diagnosed probable leukemia, and he set up a Tuesday appointment for her with a hematologist.

As he reentered Elsbeth's room, a nurse was taking her blood pressure. The stand holding the apparatus had a green sheet of paper taped to it, with "This one works" hand scrawled across the center. The nurse took her temperature and then asked about everything she'd had to drink. "One-half glass of water, two cups of orange juice, soup, cherry pop." Elsbeth had to drink $2\frac{1}{2}$ quarts of liquids every day. "Fortunately I am very thirsty. But this canned orange juice! I think it's starting to become part of my blood." The nurse left and brought back a big can of pineapple juice.

"When I woke up, it was six o'clock and all foggy," Elsbeth said. "In Switzerland, when it's foggy like that, it means fall is near—frost patterns on windows and colorful fall trees. I was surprised to see it in the first week of August. I love the fog."

It was warm. David sat by the window and turned on the air conditioner. By his shoulder was a fish made of stained glass—a blue body with yellow fins and tail, saucily suspended from a white suction cup on the window, but swimming slightly downhill. David had bought it for her in the hospital gift shop.

"I really like that fish," she told him.

"Yes, but I have a hard time seeing it swimming there in the sky," he said. "Seems funny."

"Oh, you have to use your imagination. It's perfectly blue behind him. I don't have any trouble at all."

"Well, I can't get used to it. Especially when I stand up and see him in the grass!"

Elsbeth asked him to help her sit up. She looked healthy, except for the IV taped to her arm and the bag of clear liquid—platelets—dripping slowly. No emaciated wraith, she was actually a bit overweight. "I feel like an old, crippled woman," she explained. "But after the drugs wear off, I can walk around."

The talk turned to a relative's impending divorce. Elsbeth interrupted, "But wouldn't you want to divorce me, Dave? What good am I to you, here in bed, causing nothing but problems?"

David was standing, having just turned toward her after putting his blue sports jacket on a chair. He was silent for a long, somewhat

A Weekend in August

awkward moment. There was no clever answer. She was kidding him, but she was not kidding. She was seeking affirmation, yet she knew in many ways he would be better off without her.

"I chose you. I love you, sweetheart. We're one."

He didn't have anything more to say. The reality of leukemia was harsh, and love was not a cure-all for the daily pressures. He moved close to her and kissed her.

She and David had discussed that, if the Bible is true, death is only a door to a far better life. She felt Psalm 23 was like truth for her with her ravaged bone marrow, life for her veins that flowed with life's and death's mixtures. "Though I walk through the valley of death, I will fear no evil. For Thou art with me . . . ."

But how can I leave David and the children? she agonized. *How can I accept that?* Her throat congested. *I've seen patients die,* she remembered. *As soon as they took their last breath, there was a tremendous peace. And when grandfather died, he cried out to my parents, "Someone's coming!" And he had a deep peace. No, I don't fear that. But leaving Dave. Leaving Boris and Erik and Karba . . . .*

Elsbeth did know fear: fear of the moment of actual death; of excruciating pain. *I'm scared I won't be able to breathe anymore. From the pain. I trust God. I believe. When the pain comes, I don't give up. I have no resentments. I don't feel sorry for myself that I have to lie here. But Dave has such a burden, and the children have a sick mother, and I can't be with them at such a wonderful age . . . . I must be patient, and pray for strength . . . .*

Since they were first married, they had made a conscious effort to "walk in each other's shoes"—to think through what the mate was experiencing. *Dave's role is not easy,* she thought. *Not easy at all.*

An aide brought her lunch tray. David took the cellophane from the soup bowl for her, and she ate lunch and later drank the tea. On their fourth wedding anniversary on Thursday she'd had a full, tempting tray but had taken only the bouillon. Now she nibbled on the cake. Dave ate the chicken, peas, bread, potatoes, and most of the cake.

An attractive Swiss girl about Elsbeth's age came into the room. She had a smile that seemed to engage her entire face. She was in the U.S. for a few months on a special program as a medical social worker. A native of Zürich, she had seen Elsbeth's maiden name, Zurbüchen, on the hospital registration and had immediately come to visit her. That was several days ago. Now they talked animatedly in German as David tried to follow the conversation. This girl was like a living flower from home, blossoming in the room, sensitive to Elsbeth's needs, enthusiastic about her brief visit to the States.

Then she left. "Erika called from Switzerland," Elsbeth informed David. "The children are fine." Erik, Boris, and Karba were to arrive from Switzerland Thursday with Renie, a sister-in-law. "I don't know how it will be, their getting to the house and seeing you, Dave, but no mother. I hope that will not be hard on them."

David moved closer to her bed to help her with her hair. His thumbs tangled with his fingers as he tried to replace the brown elastic band which held her hair back at the nape of her neck. Elsbeth, smiling, looked up at him as his fingers were still fumbling. "Shall I show you one more time on your finger?"

"No," he grumbled, exasperated. "I'm doing fine."

Elsbeth grabbed his pants pockets and pulled herself up on the bed a bit more. "Who called you a stubborn Norwegian?" she asked, smiling ruefully. "Yes, I know you are!"

A nurse had walked in and was writing on a pad. Hearing the remark, she asked, *"Snakker du Norsk?"* ("Do you speak Norwegian?") She was tall, very blonde, with angular but pretty features, and she was distinctly Norwegian.

"No, I'm afraid I don't," David replied. "My father does—and I wish I did."

"Well, I don't either," the nurse replied. "Just a few phrases." Then she told about the gala Sons of Norway conventions. "My husband is Irish, but he wears a button that says 'Kiss me, I'm Norwegian!' He'll take advantage of anything!" They discussed the Leif Erikson Society and the man who decorated the Leif Erikson statue. He was written up in the papers pushing the fact Columbus wasn't first. "He's even got Thanksgiving tied in with the Norwegians," the nurse was saying. "He'd prove *everything* was started by Norwegians. Hubert Humphrey is even sponsoring a bill to . . . ."

"Hubert Humphrey is Norwegian?" David asked incredulously.

A Weekend in August

"Sure!"

"Too bad. I never particularly liked him."

They were in a light mood and before long they were talking about Elsbeth's Land-Rover in Ngoshe. "It had so much play in the steering wheel," David explained, "it felt as if it weren't connected to the tie-rod."

"I wish I could go back to it—you go right through those huge holes and ruts and never feel them," Elsbeth reminisced.

"She drove over them for three years and never had an accident."

"But you should have seen me getting used to cars when I got back to Switzerland!" Elsbeth was starting to laugh. "At the airport I slammed the door on my father's Volkswagen station wagon. 'What are you doing?' my parents yelled. I had just about tipped the car over. And late one night I got out—and *slaaam!* 'It's the middle of the night! Everyone is sleeping!' my father complained. He was so upset!"

Elsbeth was laughing hard now. "But the worst was when Dad asked me if I wanted to drive. I said, 'Yes, I have to get used to it after that Land-Rover.' And I told myself I had to brake very carefully, because I used to pump the brakes hard three times on the Land-Rover. But when I came to the corner and hit the brakes, I put Dad into the windshield anyway!"

Later, a nurse came in to check Elsbeth's IV. "Will I get the blood that was ordered?" Elsbeth asked.

"No, the doctor couldn't read the numbers because the label got detached. We'll have to do that tomorrow."

Elsbeth's emotional reaction to this news caused constrictions from throat to stomach. She had been scheduled for blood eight hours ago, but an emergency open-heart surgery case had taken her pint. Now this new pint was ruined, too. All week she'd looked forward to being free of the IV on Sunday—free to walk and move without dragging the IV stand with her. If the IV slipped out at night, it would have to be restarted in scarred veins that burn and sting when probed with the needle.

"Can't you just cross match the blood?" David asked.

She told him no. He said he couldn't understand why not. She went to double-check and returned to say it was against lab regulations. They interacted some more, friendly and businesslike, with Dave getting nowhere and feeling frustrated. Finally the nurse left.

"It's a shame," David said to Elsbeth. "The blood's just sitting there."

"I really wanted to be without that IV tomorrow."

They were silent awhile. Then Elsbeth said, "Yesterday a technician came in and wanted to take blood. I knew they had to start an IV, so I asked if he could use the same hole. The answer was no, so I requested, 'Would you ask Dr. Gordin?' He reluctantly did, and Dr. Gordin came and said, 'Sure.' In fact, he said he'd draw the blood himself and send it over. He was really on my side. Most of them try, but they don't realize . . . ."

"Yes, it upsets their schedules."

They felt helpless, frustrated, as if they were treading the same rough waters. They were chips of wood in the froth.

They sat for a time with David's chair close to her bed. Between her pillow and the Maine lake scene was a tiny TV set mounted on a long, beige extender-arm. It looked like a department store "private eye" monitoring the room.

Someone had also brought a 21" portable set in for viewing President Ford's inauguration. David snapped it on as Evel Knievel was shown roaring over a line of cars on his motorcycle. Knievel then talked about his $3,000 wardrobe. A doctor described x-rays of his fractures, metal plates, and screws. Knievel then flew over the fountain at Caesar's Palace, crashing into the concrete at ninety miles per hour. In slow motion, the camera showed him sprawling, twisting, flipping, his head banging, motorcycle tumbling. Then the film clips speeded up Charlie Chaplin style as they rushed Knievel to the operating room and sang a humorous tune about putting a plate in his hip and buttoning his lip.

"I can't believe that's for real," David observed. Knievel then asked, "Are we gonna die when the time comes? Do we break through the flames? Or do we get it like anyone else?"

Marshall Efron was then shown on the screen. He was sitting, very businesslike, with a half-dozen cans in front of him and a ruler in hand. It was straight satire. At first David and Elsbeth hardly realized

A Weekend in August

it wasn't another commercial. Efron talked seriously about the critical problem of government grading of olives—giant, jumbo, extralarge. "The dictionary says giant is eminent, above others. Then there is large, mammoth, and colossal." Elsbeth began laughing but it started to hurt her.

"Please stop laughing, Dave."

David was roaring as Efron talked about supercolossal and supersupreme. "Really, Dave, please stop laughing. It's hurting me. I can't breathe." But Dave couldn't resist as Efron presented his last size—gargantuan—which was so big one olive filled the whole can.

David turned to Elsbeth. She was an odd mixture of laughter with very noticeable pain.

Visiting hours were long past. He kissed Elsbeth, then cut down the service entrance to the parking lot. His Plymouth was along the curb and he easily drove it among the stream of departing cars that snaked past the huge expanse of lawn and clumps of tall trees. David thought: *Elsbeth's temperature was up a degree. An infection would kill her. The septicemia at Temple was unbearable. Such pain. I hope that temperature doesn't stay up.*

Fifteen minutes later he pulled into the driveway. As his foot hit the front step, he heard the phone ringing. David held up his keys in the dim light, searching for the right one. He hated to pick up the phone and have it go dead. He rushed and fumbled in the dark for the keyhole, twisted, yanked the door open, and grabbed the phone in the front hall.

"Is this Dr. Christensen?" It was a woman with a decidedly Greek accent.

"Yes."

"Where have you been? I have been trying to get you all day. Did you just walk in the door?"

"Who is this please?"

"What kind of a doctor are you, anyway, that you can't be reached?"

"Who is this? Will you tell me who you are?"

Giggle.

"Elsbeth! You monkey!"

She had dialed the number, knowing he would soon be getting to the door, and she had let it ring and ring. She had called to tell him her temperature was down. And that she still happened to love him.

SUNDAY

Elsbeth was sitting in a chair, the IV taped to her arm, as David walked in at ten Sunday morning. "Hi. How are you this morning?"

"I was fine till just five minutes ago. I was walking around, straightening up the room, and looking at the plants. Then, like a bolt from the blue, this pain came—here." She made a sweeping motion from her shoulder down to her hips.

David helped her into bed. An aide came in answer to the light. Elsbeth's voice trembled and her face contorted as she asked for medication. David picked up a towel and wiped off her face.

"What is it like?" David asked. "A sharp pain?"

"No, numb. Dull. Deep down in the bones. Pressures, like I'm being paralyzed. Very hard to breathe." Her face contorted again. "Awful. Just awful pain."

"Does it come and go?"

"It just hurts like mad."

A nurse brought her some pills. Elsbeth took them, but would have preferred something more potent.

"I was so fine this morning, so happy. The pain was gone. Then it comes and it almost kills you."

David reached over and held her hand. He closed his eyes and started speaking aloud, "Lord, again we ask for Your Presence. We ask You to hear Elsbeth's cries. You knew even this would happen . . . ."

Dr. Gordin entered. "Is the pain down your lower back?"

"No, this is a new pain. But very bad. If I got up, I know I'd pass out. It's like all my blood vessels are stopped, like I'm being paralyzed."

She writhed on the bed a few inches and cried out softly.

"It feels like someone is operating on me without anesthesia."

David wiped her face and asked, "Remember that after your C-section they'd forgotten to give you a shot? How terrible that was?"

"Oh, but this is worse!"

A Weekend in August

Being operated on without anesthesia. The thought ground into David's nerve endings. *She isn't just playing with words. If I stood here watching a knife slashing through her belly or slowly severing her arm, I couldn't stand it. But all I can read is what's on her face.*

"This must have to do with my marrow. Or nerves. I don't feel it in the stomach or muscles." She asked David to help her sit up, her knees against her chin, face rigid. "It's a little better now." After sixty seconds she slid back by herself onto the pillow, stretching her legs straight, her pretty print nightgown incongruous with the pain. She tried to smile. "A Hausa can be absolutely dying," she commented, "but when someone asks how he is, it's always *lafia*—well."

Dr. Gordin, in his white coat and pants, sat with his legs crossed, patiently watching her. He was very young and had a slight mustache and thick, curly black hair. His expression was benign, concerned. "Your arm still hurt?"

"Yes."

"Your x-ray today looks better."

"Think it was an infiltrate?" David asked.

The conversation moved between the two young doctors across Elsbeth's bed: "Myeloblastic; heart murmur, grade 5; white count, 100; platelets cause clots in venous side; heparin with thrombosis; aplastic marrow." Elsbeth did not listen to the words about her body. Her eyes were on the dull green wall. "When the pain comes out of the blue," she said to them, "it's so terrible you can't describe it. So unbelievable."

The pain started to ease off, leaving her weak. Dr. Gordin left. David helped her to the sink to freshen up. She could barely stand. *Imagine this girl, who ramrodded Land-Rovers through rutted roads, needing help to apply her deodorant,* he thought. *Life changes so much.*

She had been in intense pain only about twenty minutes. His thoughts went back to Wednesday when she had been in the same kind of agony for fourteen hours. He had been sitting there joking with her Wednesday morning when the pain had suddenly hit. Shots and pills wouldn't relieve it. She'd said it was like someone going back and forth with a saw through her muscles and bones. She had been moaning terribly. Fourteen hours!

Why the pain? Why did she have to go through all this?

He'd try to cheer her up. Even now he was about to say something bright. *But who am I to urge her to cheer up? Do I say that to bring her up to me, with a smile on her face—instead of going to the depths with her? Am I just protecting myself? Am I a Job's comforter? Cheer up! I can say it but I can't experience her suffering, so I'd better shut up. I can't really share, no matter how hard I try. The pain. Leaving her children. Wondering if they'll remember her years from now. Even if the room is full of greeting cards, and people all over the world are praying for her, no one can go to her depths. She's alone.*

"Would a bath help?" he asked.

"Yes, I think so."

He helped her across the room and into the tub. She was very weak. She soaked awhile. He had difficulty helping her out. But the stimulation had helped her circulation, and she felt better.

Elsbeth had to go to the bathroom. A nurse came in to help her, and David said he'd go for a walk.

Across from Lankenau Hospital was a huge Catholic seminary, rising on a hill like a massive Michelangelo masterpiece of sixteenth century Italy. Acres of lawns rolled away from it, royal-green carpets spreading from the stately buildings. To the left was a little forest of high, old trees—oaks, ash, maple, and birch. David walked down the Lankenau lawns and across the street into the forest. He followed sandy paths half covered by weeds. *How devastated her life is,* he thought. *With her fierce maternal instincts—to be wrenched from her children!*

The path suddenly turned steeply uphill, and the trees grew taller. He could barely hear the cars on the road far below. *Maybe I'm being weak,* he thought, *trying to lean on her, sucking Elsbeth into everything on the pretext of our being one. Maybe we're too brutally frank, talking about the funeral arrangements and buying a grave next to Lois's . . . .*

At the top of the hill he came out onto the lawn of a new dormitory. He walked toward the massive buildings to the right, past the caretaker's cottage. *Back when the whole thing started, it was night-*

marish. As if I'd had $1,000 in my wallet and lost it. No! I'd grab for the pocket. Can't be lost. I'll surely find it. There's some new, glorious fact somewhere, and this whole thing will be over. But there's never been that Aaah! Found! feeling. And now we just ride with the punches. But how much can you take without hope?

He'd thought of his own death—death as release from the machine that was crushing him in its greasy gears. He even thought of suicide. *What height of irresponsibility to desert my children now, to leave Elsbeth to fight it alone! How evil were Satan's temptations.*

By now he was standing before the wide entrance to the seminary; it was lined by tall hedges and bushes for about six hundred feet. Then, at the end was a double-size statue of Christ placed in front of the stately building. The towering, robed Jesus was standing with a life-size man in a business suit crouched under His protecting arm.

David walked up close to the statue and stared at it for a while. It was impressive. The hand of Jesus was raised over the man; but somehow the marble fingers of the protective and loving God-Man had gotten knocked off.

Before David returned to Elsbeth's room, he could hear the voices. The IV had come out, and now they had to restart it for the blood which had finally arrived.

Elsbeth looked up at him, obviously frustrated that she had to go through an IV start again, especially when it could have been avoided. "Why were you gone so long?" she asked. The slight tone of disapproval in her voice communicated how she had missed him, had needed him to be there. He had mixed feelings: wanting to reassure her; yet wanting to protest that he'd had a fine walk and wanted to describe the forest and buildings.

The young intern had trouble with the IV. For the next hour David moved in and out of her room, not wanting to make him nervous by staring, but not wanting to desert Elsbeth, either. Time after time the doctor failed to get it started. The needle stung in her scarred tissue. Frustration rasped at her nerves and finally she started crying. David held her hand. The pain was coming back, and she needed a shot, but they were too busy trying to stick her.

She looked over at the young, frustrated doctor and smiled at him.

"I don't want you to think I mind your sticking me. It's okay," she said to him.

She's a precious patient, David was thinking. He was so frustrated and knew he—or Elsbeth herself—could have started the IV without trouble. Yet he couldn't keep butting in. He remembered trying to do everything himself at Erik's birth. He had had to induce Elsbeth's labor, and when she began to have spasms, he learned the emotional pitfalls of treating one's own wife. Now, after having operated on Elsbeth twice, he knew it was too emotional, too pressured for him to carry all the responsibility.

In some ways this was worse. So many small things added to her discomfort. Now the young doctor was sticking her in the foot, trying to get at a vein, and David felt like smashing the IV bottle against the wall. "The trying of your faith worketh patience," he mentally repeated again and again. Sometimes both he and Elsbeth felt like canceling all this—go home to die. He could give her pain medications. Yet, she'd already lived almost a year. She'd experienced Switzerland, her children growing, their new home, witnessing for Christ. How could they reject the possibility of another year, whatever the agony?

Finally, after eleven attempts, the intern gave up and called the resident. Dr. Margaret Shep then successfully started the IV on the first try.

David sat at the foot of her bed after the doctors left. She'd had a shot, but her body was still agitated. "What a day!" she murmured flatly. It was supposed to have been a relaxed Sunday without an IV—before the new chemotherapy and its resulting nausea. Why did this day have to be so bad? Was God using it, perhaps, in someone's life? Would someone be drawn closer to God through it? Were Elsbeth's pains the spiritual birth pangs for someone else? Or was there some other purpose of God? Dave was asking her if she thought so, and at first she did not answer.

"Do you think so?" he asked again. Finally she nodded a perfunctory assent. It was an assent only, not an endorsement of the idea. God's using her as a tool? As a "vessel"? Perhaps. But one could be foolishly simplistic about specifics, dangerously applying cause and effect. *We can't see God's blueprint,* David thought. *The gems of*

A Weekend in August

meaning are not scattered on top of the earth to finger and examine.

Her heart was beating rapidly. He could see from where he sat the double-rate shaking of her chest under her blue, flowered nightgown. "Do you feel your heart beating like that?" he asked.

Her reply was so quiet he had to read her lips to catch it. "Yes," she said. "But it doesn't matter. It will stop soon."

She was not asking for pity or playing a role. It was a bland statement, a resignation. How could one keep fighting when her body acted like this? The inevitable squeezed upon her like a giant hand with steel, penetrating fingers.

The day blended into a tedious gray. Tedium. Tedium. Elsbeth endured one kind, lying there with constant procedures and pain; David's was another kind of tedium, sitting, waiting, and trying to reassure and show love with so few ways available to do it.

He had promised a friend he'd drive him to the airport. It seemed an interruption now, yet he knew it would feel good to get away.

"Don't get lost, Dave," she told him, only half kidding. Philadelphia suburbs have been termed the most confusing labyrinth in America. David, who prided himself on the unerring map in his head, had on occasion driven in circles for up to an hour. "If you get lost, ask somebody. Don't just drive around," she taunted. "You're so stubborn about that."

"Asking doesn't always work either. People give you directions and you end up *really* lost."

"Don't get hurt," she added, with an implied *hurry back* in the inflections. He was her only pipeline to the outside world.

As he entered his car, he felt the tension move with him. Even away from it, that hospital room was like his car. It encased him. It was around and under and in front of him, capturing him thoroughly as he used hands and eyes and feet to go through the motions of life. Yet he was coping. At his office nurses would say, "I don't know how you do it, Dr. Christensen." "I'd be a basket case." "You show such interest in the patients and smile and even laugh with them." "You're so strong." He liked to hear that and fought against his liking it. He had to fight against becoming a living martyr and enjoying the status. He had to pray against pride's seeping in through an insidious new door. He would catch himself doing things for the effect they would have on others. His task was to be himself—not a living object lesson—and not to relate to God with secondary motives. *In my most holy moments, I'm still an unworthy sinner,* he thought as he wheeled through the dozens of turns and angles and confusing signs he'd only recently figured out.

He maneuvered around the construction at Philadelphia International Airport and dropped his friend off under the TWA sign. Then, he waved and moved into the slow line of cars again.

Lankenau Hospital. It was still with him. He had heard the cliché of "feeling like a yoyo at the end of a string." But now it took on a jarring meaning, as if any nearby telephone cord were the string. It was umbilical—always dangling close to his belly, always ready to jolt his stomach acids into quick action by its jangling announcement of a new crisis.

It is one thing to face the shock of death. But it is another thing to live hour after hour, day after day, with death—always having it attached firmly to you. In the office, at home with the kids, or wherever, he was constantly thinking: *Does Elsbeth need me now? Did an IV slip? Will she suddenly writhe on the bed, and, perhaps, even die before I get there? Will she die alone and wanting me so much—maybe even calling, "Where is he? Dave! Dave!"?*

9

The Light

DOWNHILL

David stood at Elsbeth's bedside pumping blood by hand into a tiny little vein on her wrist. He had been doing this all day because she had no unscarred big veins.

It was Saturday, September 28. Elsbeth had been in the hospital nine weeks. She now had hepatitis, with jaundice and a fever. She had almost no resistance to infection. Yet she was in remission . . . the cancer cells had been purged!

Weeks ago she had told David, "I can't take it anymore. I just want to die." Instead of improving, her condition had gotten worse. Every time they felt they could bear no more, something new marauded their spirits: an eye infection, abscesses in her lymph nodes which required surgery, painful hemorrhoids, a minor operation that failed. She had taken prednisone to cut her fever and woke up every two hours at night with cold sweats. Although she was covered with three blankets, she still felt freezing cold and was so soaked she could wring out her nightgown. This happened night after night, for five nights.

"Think of what the Vietnam prisoners went through," Elsbeth commented now as David's hand squeezed in and out, pumping the blood. "Stuck in boxes. Beaten. Tortured. Sick. No hope. They suffered worse."

"So many people are praying for a miracle," David responded. "Why don't we see it? Yet God is giving you the strength to bear all this. That's a miracle."

Elsbeth needed not only fortitude—but patience—to withstand the huge disappointments and, also, the little episodes. "Nurse, I have trouble sleeping with the light on all night," Elsbeth had said softly one evening. The response: the light must stay on. In the operating room, Elsbeth had been lying for twenty minutes covered only by a sheet, freezing in the air conditioning. "May I have a blanket?"

"No, young lady," a nurse had replied sarcastically. "We don't have any wool blankets up here." The words made her feel like meat on a cart.

She met infuriating incompetence which caused unnecessary pain. Most workers were efficient and caring. The trouble was, she and David knew too much about medicine and noticed lapses and bad decisions.

Even the best times were clouded. Two weeks ago David had bundled her up in a wheelchair to take her outside for the first time. As David got her to the door, she didn't want to go out. "Why not?" David asked. Elsbeth looked up at him: "Why does everybody want me to go outside? Why does the doctor say, 'Take her out!'? Are they all thinking I'm dying, and this will be my last time?" But they did go out and enjoyed the fall colors, the wide, hilly lawns, and clear air. She began to understand the stories of prisoners who came to think of their cells as home and wouldn't want to leave. She felt safe here in her room with her pictures, mobiles, and walls full of bright cards.

Elsbeth watched David. She had to lie perfectly still as he pumped the blood. *Why do you do all this if I am going to die?* It seemed absurd to leave her little family so soon—who would be Mother to Erik, Boris, and Karba? She could hardly stand being away from them in the hospital, let alone the thought of leaving them forever. For some time now Elsbeth thought she knew the future. Almost the same month they had learned of Elsbeth's leukemia, Carol—the girl David had "given up" years ago as a student—had called with the sad news that her husband, Mike, a jet-fighter pilot, had been killed when his ejection seat had exploded. From the day of the phone call, the news seemed to be an omen to Elsbeth. Was God's timing involved here? Carol had three little girls. David would need a wife. They had dated seriously in the past. Both Mike and Carol had re-

The Light

mained David's close friends. "I think it's natural you should think of Carol," Elsbeth had admitted to David one day. "I feel she is the one to become your wife. After I die you could take the children to the Poconos, then fly out to California to see if she's the one." It had been very hard for Elsbeth to say that. But she wanted to be realistic and to free David to make a life for himself.

David had listened. Her words made him uneasy, but he agreed to think about it. As he did, however, he found it a trap. When his mind would explore the possibility of marrying Carol and his wish to swoop up her children and protect and love them, he found it a means of mental escape from Elsbeth's trauma. He felt Satan starting to use it against him, that it could become a form of mental adultery to make such plans. Elsbeth was still his wife. He loved Elsbeth! It was God's job to care for Carol and her little girls. He had gotten on his knees: "Lord, Elsbeth is my wife. I'm going to love *her*," he had pledged. "This is wrong for me to even think about Carol."

Elsbeth watched David squeezing the little tube. "Dave, I really think you are going to marry Carol," she confided, not knowing of his earlier prayer.

David looked at her steadily, his hand still pumping. "No, Elsbeth," he insisted, "I'm not going to marry Carol. You're my wife. It's *you* I love. I'm not going to think about marrying Carol. I'm not going to give you up! I'm going to keep on praying that you'll get well!"

But her signs were not good. This morning they had learned her white blood count had dropped lower, which meant her resistance was almost nil. Every time she would try to get up, she would faint.

Finally the blood was pumped. David turned on "The New Land," a TV story about Norwegian immigrants. Elsbeth felt better and enjoyed the program. Perhaps her symptoms were mostly from the hepatitis. That was old hat—she could lick hepatitis. David read from Philippians, and Elsbeth drowsed off to sleep. She woke up in a funny position, and both laughed about it. They began to feel lighthearted because she felt better. David went on to read the whole Book of Philippians to her.

David went home that night relaxed, thankful she was feeling better. But during the night she called; she was in terrible pain again. At eight the next morning she woke up shaking. She called David again; she was shivering from so much pain. He could hardly recognize her voice.

David arrived to see everyone in whites around her bed. A nurse was cranking her feet up. Elsbeth was shaking. By the afternoon Elsbeth said, "Dave, I can't stand it anymore. My head is pounding." He took her temperature and went and told the nurse it was 106°. The nurses were changing shifts and no one came, so David went back to the desk. "You've got to do something. That temp can't go much higher."

A nurse came into her room with a basin of alcohol and water. She put the air conditioner on, then laid big, wet towels on her body. Elsbeth felt she was freezing, though her body was burning. After three-quarters of an hour, the fever had not come down. David decided to put her in a tub of lukewarm water, which to Elsbeth felt like icy torture. He brought the fever down to 103°.

David almost carried her back to the bed. When he had gotten her settled, she said to him, "Dave, I feel absolutely awful. I've never felt this way before. I really feel I'm dying." They prayed then, and Elsbeth asked the Lord to give her peace.

She was suffering from septic shock. Her fever went back up to 106°. She was turning purple, since there was bleeding into her skin. They put her into an oxygen tent.

By the evening she had been given so many fluids that she was thrown into congestive heart failure. However, the heart pumped on.

By Monday morning her chest was gurgling, and they gave massive amounts of diuretics to flush out the fluids. Her face was swollen and purple. She had become nearly deaf from the high doses of antibiotics, so that David had to shout for her to hear. She could barely see. Her breathing and pulse were rapid. She had developed pneumonia and was usually in a coma.

On Tuesday Dr. Gabuzda asked if David had noticed anything strange about Elsbeth's emotional state. "Yes," he replied as they stood in the hall outside her room. "It's just not the same Elsbeth. My Elsbeth is gone. She's like a mummy. She doesn't cry, she doesn't have feeling." The doctor agreed that the trauma—the smashing of hope—was making her psychotic. He was willing to morphinize her for David's sake, so she'd be sleeping all the time.

The Light

But David didn't want that. Her deafness was probably irreversible. She was unconscious most of the time, and when she did awake, she was disoriented, talking about getting sand into the sandbox. There was very little hope. Yet to shut her off . . . .

Life outside made demands on him. He had to make some house calls. He realized it was October 1, Karba's tenth birthday, and he hadn't bought a present for her. Worse than that, they had been promising her a birthday party for a long time, but now, nothing had been arranged. He hated to disappoint her. He had asked Karba weeks ago, "If you could wish for anything in the whole world for your birthday, what would you want?" Karba's reply was quick, "For my mommy to come home from the hospital." David knew he couldn't produce that, but he wished he could have delivered on the party.

David went out and bought a present, then went home and took Karba and "Nana" out to dinner. David's grandmother, Nana, was staying with them to cook the meals. David then dropped Nana off at home to get a birthday cake ready, while he took Karba to the hospital.

Elsbeth broke through her coma and even smiled a bit as she handed Karba the little present and a card. Just then, to David's surprise, a group of nurses came in and sang happy birthday to Karba before she opened her present. Elsbeth never heard the rest of the song. David tried to awaken her, but she barely opened her eyes.

They said good-bye and drove home. Just as David pulled up at the sidewalk in front of their home, he noticed three little figures—two girls and a boy—walking down the street toward them. They yelled out, "Happy birthday, Karba!"

The children started toward her with presents, but David interrupted, "Why don't you come in and give them to her?" They got into the foyer and were taking off their coats as David nodded to Nana. She lighted the cake, and when Karba turned around her eyes widened in complete surprise and pleasure.

"Well, come on, kids, come in and have some cake," David invited. As they sat around the dining-room table, he was amazed. The Myers children had gotten into their minds to bring her a present, and they showed up just as David and Karba arrived for cake. Now, she was having a wonderful party. He hadn't even prayed about this. The whole experience gave him a buoyancy. *If the Lord,* he thought, *looks after Karba for such a little thing—but such a big thing to her—wouldn't He look after Elsbeth?*

GOOD-BYE TO THE BOYS

David watched Elsbeth's unconscious form on the bed. It was Wednesday. He had just learned she had interstitial pneumonia, a grave form which meant infection of the lung membranes themselves. She was on all the antibiotics available, and David knew that to survive, her body had to repel the infection, but it had no white cells to do so.

Her eyes opened. He reached his hand into the oxygen tent and held hers. Her mouth was caked and her tongue swollen. A nurse came in, and David watched Elsbeth's eyes fix on her. It took a long, long time, but she moved her head to look up as the nurse adjusted the IV. Elsbeth forced a smile at her. Almost before the smile was finished, she lapsed into unconsciousness.

Suddenly she woke up again. In a weak monotone, gasping for breath, she rasped out one word at a time: "Dave, am I dying?"

David listened with all his powers, barely deciphering her words. He had to shout his response over the noise of the machinery: "Do you think you're dying?"

There was a long pause as Elsbeth fought to hold on to reality. Finally her thick, dry tongue painfully formed the words, "I don't know." Her response gave him hope; if she were dying, she would probably sense it.

An aide came in with water. After she left David shouted, "Are you ready to die?"

She took a full ten seconds to gasp out each individual word: "Yes, I am ready."

"Well, if you do die," he said gently, "the first question I want you to ask when you see Jesus is *Why?* Ask Him why, and He'll tell you, and then you'll be happy." David was surprised that even in this conversation she smiled.

Wednesday seemed to be a day when people came to pay their

last respects. Elsbeth gained consciousness again, and David told her that Wali and Trud, her brother and his wife, were coming from Switzerland. Each time after that when she'd open her eyes she'd ask, "Are they really coming?"

"Yes, they're on the plane now," David would reply, glad to give her something to look forward to. But he had seen a lot of people die. He feared she would not last till they arrived.

Elsbeth sensed everyone knew she was dying. Nurses would come, smile, give their injections, be friendly, but Elsbeth mused, "I know exactly what you think when I see you coming." She felt like she was almost on the other side already, especially in the oxygen tent. If someone looked in from the outside, the heavy plastic which hung loosely around her distorted their faces into long oddities with bulging eyes. Sometimes when the lights were on, and they were walking around, she could hardly stand it. She felt almost like a ghost separated from real people. When the humidifier inside the tent would go off it made a loud *brrrrr* noise. Her vision was distorted; she saw something floating. She refused to be touched, the pain was so intense. If the tent was opened for just ten minutes she would turn blue. She felt wet and cold from the humidity.

A little after nine o'clock she awoke and looked at David sitting by her bed. He was shocked that she was bright and alert, even though her words came slowly and laboriously: "Dave, I have just one question to ask you."

David thought she was going to resume the conversation about death. "Sure, what is it?"

"Don't you think I should see the children?"

David was taken aback. "Have you been thinking of that before?"

"Yes."

He felt guilty. Obviously she hadn't been able to express her thoughts, and he had not wanted to create more problems for her. He called his aunt in the Poconos and said he didn't know if Elsbeth would live till morning. Could they bring Erik and Boris right away? Then he sat down by the window and watched the airplanes in the sky. Elsbeth was unconscious again, but when Wali and Trud arrived, she did wake up enough to know they were there. She smiled and greeted them, then drifted off.

A little after midnight David carried Erik, and his Uncle John carried little Boris into the room. Both boys were wide awake as if it were morning. Elsbeth woke up and smiled passively. David sat Erik on the bed, and the three-year-old took hold of her hand and smiled from ear to ear. "Mommy, I love you," he stated boldly. Then as he watched his mother's emotionless face, he asked, "Mommy, you know what?"

Elsbeth very slowly focused on his face and said, "What?"

"Mommy, you're sad."

Elsbeth just kept looking at him, unable to respond. David asked his son, "Erik, why is Mommy sad?"

"I know why Mommy is sad. She doesn't have Erik with her in the hospital." Then his face stretched into his big grin again and he repeated, "Mommy, I love you." David was amazed. *If I had planned with Erik in advance, he couldn't have done better,* he thought.

David then tried to put the younger Boris down to kiss his mommy, but he wanted to hug her and jump on the bed. "Mommy *boo-boo*. Mommy *boo-boo*," he exclaimed: it was his phrase for injury.

Erik knew, from former visits, that candy was kept in a can. He began asking for it. David took out the saltwater taffy and on a whim handed it to Elsbeth. She forced her fingers to slowly, mechanically unwrap the paper. Erik watched with anticipation. Finally she succeeded and reached out to put it into Erik's mouth. David was surprised she had the willpower to do all this, or the awareness to even know Erik had a mouth. Then, just as Erik was going to take a bite, she pulled it away to tease him a little, brought it to her own mouth and bit off a piece. Erik's eyes widened, then Elsbeth handed Erik the other half.

He chewed it down, and by this time Boris had eaten his, too. Then the boys kissed their mother good-bye. She watched them go. She had previously felt no peace about leaving them, but she had prayed and prayed, turning it over to the Lord, asking Him to care for her children. And now He had given her His peace.

THURSDAY, OCTOBER 3

On Thursday morning the doctors gave Elsbeth morphine. She wished they'd done so earlier, for all night she had struggled to get

The Light

her breath. David sat by her bed, watching her fever rise despite antibiotics. Few people came. She was purple, and her face was puffed. David felt it was a deathwatch. Once in a while she would awaken and ask if "Mueti," her mother, was really coming from Switzerland, and David would respond, "Yes, she's on the plane right now."

At seven that evening, Dr. Gabuzda, chief of Hematology, took her blood pressure, pulse, and temperature and listened to her lungs. Then he came to David at the door to the room. "Her blood pressure is stable. She's through the septic shock. The problem is her ventilation."

"Have you ever seen anyone with this diagnosis pull out of it?"

The doctor looked directly into David's eyes and admitted, "No. I've never seen anyone recover who had interstitial pneumonia like this. Of course, there could be a first time—I don't want to take away all hope. But I've never seen anyone this far gone recover. Basically, the battle is now yours." The doctor looked David in the eyes again and repeated the statement. "The battle is now yours."

David didn't ask him to elaborate. He understood him to say that her fight was over, but that his was just beginning. He thanked him, then sat down by her bed again and reached for a writing tablet. His mind was whirling with thoughts, and he only hoped she would live long enough to see her mother. He started to rough out a prayer letter.

"Dear faithful friends," he began, "This evening, after nearly ten weeks of hospitalization, my dear Elsbeth went to dwell in the presence of our dear Lord Jesus. Elsbeth did not want to go at this time. She felt needed. She wanted to take care of her husband and her children. She did not understand why the Lord should give her only four years of married life. Yet Elsbeth, even on her death bed said, 'I want only the Lord's will.'"

As he was writing this, Elsbeth woke up and looked at him. He was startled and amazed at the clarity in her eyes. He smiled at her and then zipped open the oxygen tent. "Elsbeth, can you see what tie I'm wearing?" She nodded. "Do you recognize it?" he asked. "This is the tie you gave me, and I'm wearing it." She smiled. She had often made humorous remarks about his not wearing it, and he would respond that its darker colors made it a winter tie for a heavier suit. "You see," he added, "I do wear it. Thank you for giving it to me."

She smiled again and grabbed the tie and pulled him a little way into the oxygen tent. David kissed her. Elsbeth kissed him back. Slowly she asked, word by word, "Dave, do you really think I'm dying?"

"Yes."

"Who says? Does Dr. Gabuzda?"

"They say it is very serious. There's hope, if you start making white cells; but you've had all the treatments, and your fever is up." She nodded at that. David told her that he had gone out a few hours ago and bought a grave lot next to Lois's and that he'd arranged the funeral—the casket would be in their home. "Is that okay? Is this what you want?" Elsbeth agreed it was, and then David asked, "Do you have any pain?"

"No."

"Are you comfortable?"

"Yes."

"Do you think you are dying?"

"I don't know," she responded in her feeble voice. It was a great effort for her to talk, and David had to almost shout because of the constant blowing, the noises of the machines, and her near deafness."

"Are you sad?" he asked.

"No."

"Do you have peace?"

"Yes," she said with assurance.

"I do, too," David said. "I love you, Elsbeth."

"I love you, too, Dave."

David was amazed she was staying clear so long. "I was just reading some of your old letters," he shouted at her. "One you wrote to me when I had the flu was that the greatest gift would be our getting better and our walking through the leaves together as a family. That's what I hope for us now." He paused, then said, "God loves us and will take care of each of us, Elsbeth."

"I know."

The Light

He thought a moment, then said what he wasn't sure he should bring up. "Elsbeth, I never had the chance to say good-bye to Lois. Will you greet her for me?"

She nodded, then lapsed back into unconsciousness.

David sat down again and felt a restful peace within. But as he kept thinking, a conflict began. Had he talked to her about the funeral arrangements and Lois just to get it off his chest? Was he using Elsbeth? Would this take away her fight? Was he selfish? He sensed he needed Elsbeth's spirit with him in what he would have to do in the next few days, to know she agreed with him. "Lord," he prayed, "don't let this in any way hurt Elsbeth. Help me to do and say only what will glorify You. Take away my selfishness. And take Elsbeth quickly, without pain." But his prayer didn't solve his feeling of grief. He thought of opening up the drawers at home and seeing the Goyesca soap she loved so much. What would he do with that now? What would he do with her clothes?

David and Elsbeth had often talked about miracles. How would they recognize one? You can always explain away almost any event with medical and scientific terms. How would other persons be convinced God had touched Elsbeth miraculously. As he sat there he thought, *If ever God is to act distinctively—if ever we could be convinced of a miracle—it would be now. There's no human hope. She's almost dead already.*

He rose to adjust the oxygen tent and noticed a little card on the table with Jeremiah 17:14 printed in German. He couldn't read it, so he looked it up in The Living Bible:

"Lord, you alone can heal me, you alone can save, and my praises are for you alone."

The verse jolted him. He was reminded that only God can heal, whether through medicine or supernatural means. And this was the night God could prove it.

David began to feel strongly convicted that this was not the time to sit around writing letters as if Elsbeth were already dead. This was a time to be talking to God!

He began to pray again fervently: that she would be healed; and just as fervently that she would be relieved of pain; and that her mother would get to see her. His prayers were not that different from previous ones, but the verses of Scripture led him away from grief into a positive prayer attitude and a new peace.

Dr. Constable, his associate, came in. David had spoken to him that morning, and he had agreed that he didn't see how Elsbeth could recover. They had talked about her death, and David had exclaimed, "The whole thing is, I'm just going to miss her!"

Dr. Constable's reply had warmed David deeply, "Well," he said, "there is no one who knows her who will not miss her."

Now he shared with his partner his thoughts and his prayer that he and Elsbeth could walk together in those leaves again. As they talked both of them realized how contradictory their real attitudes were—her feet were stiffening in a foot-drop position. "Here we are praying for her to be healed," David said, "and what if she recovers and can't walk because of her feet?" So they rigged up a makeshift footboard and put it on her.

The phone rang. It was a Swiss Air agent, calling from Boston. Mueti would be an hour late getting into Philadelphia. David thanked him and was just about to hang up the phone when he saw Elsbeth's eyes looking at him out of the oxygen tent. "Elsbeth, can you hear me?" he shouted. She nodded her head. "Just a minute," he said to the Swiss Air man, "Is Mrs. Zürbuchen still there?" David put the phone into the tent with Elsbeth, and she talked with her mother for a full minute, then lapsed back into unconsciousness.

David continued praying. Shortly after midnight Mueti came into the room. She was tired and nervous. Elsbeth awoke, then reached up and put her left hand hard on the back of Mueti's neck, pulling her down and kissing her. But Mueti looked at her eyes, and they seemed almost fixed . . . . She was still purple.

David left the special-duty nurse in charge as he left with Mueti. He was deeply aware of God. He had a strange feeling as he went to sleep that night that Elsbeth was going to be all right.

LEAVES AND WOLVES

The next morning, Friday, Elsbeth woke up for a full hour and talked with Wali, Trud, and Mueti. They were stunned. That afternoon, her white count came back at two thousand, almost ten times

The Light

as high as yesterday. By evening, Dr. Gabuzda was telling David he couldn't allow himself to be excited, but he was pleased and hopeful that Elsbeth would be with them when he returned after the weekend.

Saturday her white count was three thousand, and by Monday morning, Dr. Gabuzda returned to find Elsbeth not only alive, but decidedly better. He came up to David, after examining her, and bubbled over with enthusiasm. "I just can't believe it. It must be divine intervention. I called in last night, and they told me she was better, but I had no idea she looked this good. I almost can't believe it—I told you I had never seen anyone in her condition pull through. Of course, we don't have the results of her latest bone marrow . . . ."

David thanked the doctor, then walked in and asked Elsbeth what he had said to her. He had told her, "You know you were gravely ill. For your case, the doctors don't get the credit. No question about it."

As they were talking, Elsbeth's surgeon came in. "I just can't believe it," he told her. "After a few days of my being away, look at how you look! If that's the case, I'm going to go away for another month!"

They talked on and David commented, "I believe God works in natural ways, but He works."

"He sure worked this time," the surgeon affirmed.

Other doctors called it a miracle, too. David and Elsbeth believed it was precisely that. Not a healing—for she probably still had leukemia—but a miracle. Doctors referred to her as "our most amazing patient."

From then on, it was recovery, inch by inch. A week later she could barely move her legs, but then her left leg regained mobility. Two days after she first got into a chair David told her, "Now you're going to stand up." She protested firmly that she couldn't, for each new step seemed impossible. She wouldn't give David an inch as she tearfully argued for ten minutes.

"The least you could do is try," David insisted. She hesitated a little, and he saw he had won. Yet he felt guilty that he had dominated her. "How?" she asked.

David got his arms under her and helped her up. Before he could even straighten out, she was off. Step. Step. Step. She was walking around the bed. David almost tripped over the chair as he tried to rush after her. Elsbeth was not just standing, but walking—and throwing her head back, laughing, laughing, and then crying, and then laughing and laughing! She just couldn't believe she was walking again! She lay down on the bed and then got up to walk around the bed in the other direction.

Three weeks after the crisis, David was driving her home. As they pulled into the driveway they saw a few leaves left on the trees and in the yard, but David had to carry her over them and into the house. He helped her walk into the living room where she collapsed on the chair and rested. She loved this room with the stone fireplace. Above the fireplace hung a painting of Jesus touching a patient in bed while the doctor and nurse looked on.

After talking for a while, David turned on the phonograph, selecting a record they had played in the hospital. The first song was "The Hiding Place."

> In a time of sorrow, in a time of grief
> There is a hiding place, to give relief.
> In a time of weakness, in a time of fear
> There is a hiding place, where God is near.

And then they listened to the second song:

> Through it all. . . .
> Through it all. . . .
> I've learned to trust in Jesus
> I've learned to trust in God.

Shortly before Thanksgiving, David and Elsbeth drove with their children to a little park three minutes away from their home. Oak trees stood tall over a trickle of a creek; there were crackly leaves

---

Excerpts from "The Hiding Place" are used by permission. Words and Music by Bryan Jeffery Leech. © Copyright 1972, 1973 by Gentry Publications, Tarzana, CA 91356. International Copyright Secured. All rights reserved.

Excerpts from "Through It All" by Andrae Crouch are © Copyright 1971 by Manna Music, Inc., 2111 Kenmere Ave., Burbank, CA 91504. International Copyright Secured. All Rights Reserved. Used by Permission.

The Light

spread over the steep hills and gullies. They put Boris in a swing with a bar to hold him securely. David climbed to the top of the slide where Erik was wondering if he should let go or not; he zoomed down with his boy in his lap. Then David ran and ran and ran—with Erik running beside him—across the creek and up a hill and down, faster and faster.

Elsbeth stood watching, smiling. She was still bothered with foot drop. She could still not see perfectly. She wondered why the Lord hadn't let her die when she was so near death. She had been ready—she had given up David, and the children, and life itself. Was God playing cat and mouse with her? *I almost can't stand it!* she thought. She would cry with the frustrations of living in her house yet not being able to be wife and mother and homemaker. She trembled at the thought of going through the hospital way of death again, at giving up her loved ones all over again.

Yet here she was, enjoying the laughter of her children and husband. She was deeply thankful. What a crisp, invigorating day! How joyous to be out here! In a way, wasn't everyone like her—suffering from a fatal disease that would kill sooner or later? She might die tomorrow. But so might David or anyone.

Dave came thundering back, winded, the exercise giving him a warm, animal sensation. He wished he could be out here with his family more often. He looked at his wife. He had said to her during the worst times, "I don't think we're puppets on the end of a string, trying to smile. God is not just playing games."

Our hope is as big as God is, David thought. He couldn't answer all the whys, but he trusted God. He and Elsbeth had discussed the wolves in the movie, *Dr. Zhivago*—they'd always been out there howling, waiting. Just as David and Elsbeth would reach for respite, for happiness, they'd hear the wolves.

THE WEDDING

During Christmas week, Carol called David and Elsbeth from Washington, D.C. She was about to be married! She wanted to know if Elsbeth was feeling well enough to be her matron of honor at the wedding the following Saturday.

Elsbeth was flabbergasted. She still had trouble walking and seeing properly. How could she participate in a wedding, just six days from now, in a huge church, with hundreds of onlookers? Furthermore, she had never even met Carol. What kind of gown would be chosen for her? The idea filled Elsbeth with anxiety. She didn't know if she could walk properly . . . but, at last, she agreed.

Around noon Saturday they arrived in Bethesda, Maryland, and entered the pastor's split-level home where the participants were preparing for the wedding. The first persons David noticed as he walked in were four-year-old Christy and Corrie, age one. He could distinctly see both Carol and Mike in their faces. Little Corrie, who to David looked more like Mike, came up to him and climbed into his arms. David hugged her. She snuggled in close and seemed quite content to sit there in his lap. He thought of his good friend Mike and of his past musings that perhaps he would be daddy to this little Corrie, and to Cheryl, and Christy. The thoughts mixed crazily in his mind and emotions. God in His Providence had not made him Christy's dad, nor had He let Mike stay with them. However, He had provided a new father. It gave David a strange, bittersweet ache.

Elsbeth, feeling quite well, was sitting with Karba on the couch. On Karba's calendar at home Elsbeth would draw a happy face or a sad face to indicate if she'd been "naughty or nice" that day. The entire December calendar had filled up with happy faces, so bringing Karba to Washington was her reward. They sat there in the chaos of pastor's kids and Carol's kids and preparations, with Corrie sitting contentedly on David's lap. Then Carol came in with six-year-old Cheryl. Coming up the steps, she saw Elsbeth and immediately threw her arms around her and enthusiastically hugged her.

That afternoon Elsbeth found, much to her relief, that the gown waiting for her fit perfectly. They were supposed to arrive at the church at six-thirty. A few minutes after six Elsbeth went to help Carol and found her in the shower, shouting past the spray and giving orders to the girls about what to wear. Elsbeth thought the situation quite humorous and she started helping. Carol then emerged in her slip and combed the girls' hair. It was swept up, with curls hanging below their ears. The girls' dresses were much like their mother's

The Light

—lace on top, and a flower belt with hanging loops under the bodice, and flowers around the neck.

"I don't want to wear this dress!" Christy suddenly declared. "I hate it. It itches. Mommy, take it off!" She was crying and going on and on, struggling against the dress as her mother tried to pull it down over her head. "I don't want the dress. I don't want to go to church. I don't want a new daddy." The four-year-old was fiercely adamant, and it was getting alarmingly late.

Carol bent down to her little daughter and, putting one arm around her, said, "Come listen, Christy. You and Cheryl have been praying for a daddy, and you know, this is a very happy day. God has answered your prayers. Our daddy knows we have a wedding today. He can see us, and he wants us to be happy, for this is a wonderful day. Now, will you please cooperate and help?" Carol kneeled there looking at her daughter quietly for a few seconds, then added, "Christy, I love you *very* much. You know that, don't you?" Then she hugged her very tightly.

After that, the little girls behaved beautifully. David drove the four participants to Fourth Presbyterian Church, then slipped off with Karba to find a seat near the front of the church. The organ was playing. The people were already seated. Elsbeth looked down the long, long aisle to the burning candles at the front. She watched the little girls standing patiently, like models for Hallmark cards, all bedecked in their flowers. Little Corrie was in a babysitter's arms, taking her bottle. *Corrie will never remember this, of course,* Elsbeth thought. *John will always be her daddy.* Elsbeth couldn't keep the other thoughts from crowding in: *In a few years from now, would Boris remember Elsbeth? Would Erik?* Nevertheless, watching Carol and realizing how God had provided for her filled Elsbeth with gratitude. She had worried so much about David and the children. But here was God providing for Carol's children. Carol, so beautiful in her flowers, must have been feeling wildly mixed emotions. Yet here was God in the middle of them—not just in the outward circumstances, but in Carol's sensing His presence and His power in her life. *Surely the Lord loves David's and my children just as much.*

They had been waiting for almost fifteen minutes. Finally, the pastor and John came out at the front. Elsbeth took her first step, feeling strong and sure of herself—the first time in almost half a year that she was wearing regular shoes. She paced herself very slowly, thinking of the little girls behind her. The shoes were tight; she had to watch each motion. The candles in the distance burned brightly. Elsbeth had to squint to see them clearly, but as she did, the soft lights diffused into sparkling beads, like an otherworldly dawn. It gave her a weird sensation as she walked slowly toward the candles while the organ played and the eyes of the congregation followed her. She knew David and Karba were sitting out there somewhere. It seemed odd that she should have to walk alone, all alone—painfully alone—up the aisle while David and Karba simply watched. *Will it be this way at my funeral?* she wondered as she slowly made her way forward. *Is the one who dies present, somehow, and walking forward like this to meet Jesus—as the others simply sit and mourn? Maybe I don't have much more time.* The light from the candles was a lovely, colorful invitation, beckoning her forward to life, to light, to a warm welcome. Yet her loved ones could not walk with her, could not be absorbed into the light with her.

David watched her slowly coming down the aisle. She walked without a limp for the first time. Her glasses were gone. Her black hair was full of chrysanthemums and roses. He wanted to take a picture of her, but his eyes were teared, and he didn't want to distract from the bride. She was *his* bride! It was as if the Lord were giving her to him all over again. Just a few months before she had been lying utterly devastated by disease—with no hope. Now she looked more beautiful than ever as she walked gracefully in front of the little flower girls. Perhaps the Lord really was restoring her to him as wife and mother and homemaker. At the very least, He seemed to have given them this wedding as a gift, as an assurance He really did care.

David wondered what Elsbeth was thinking. Here she was witnessing what might happen to David in a year or so. Elsbeth was walking in front of a bride who was exchanging her love for one man to someone new. *It must be God's grace in Carol's heart,* David thought. *A marvel, but it hurts to think of it. That God would substitute another person for Elsbeth is a terrible concept.*

David watched his lover near the candles. He was uplifted with

The Light

hope, although he was distressingly saddened at the same instant. Here was his bride. *Lord, keep the wolves away!* he prayed. *But whatever You do—though You slay us—yet we will trust You.*

Getting closer to the candles, Elsbeth still tightened her eyes against the light. She loved the stunningly beautiful pink hues spattered with pinpricked rays of reds and purples. David and Karba were still unseen somewhere behind her. She stood beyond them before the light, solitary in her thoughts.

Christy and Cheryl came up, and then Carol. After the exchange of rings and vows, they knelt. A solo was sung and John, the groom, beamed happily. Yet the pastor and best man, thinking of the little girls and all the events, wept, and the pastor had trouble speaking. *Joy out of grief.*

Life! Hope! Joy! It comes to us in such strange packages, Elsbeth thought. *But God does not play cat and mouse with us. In so many, many ways I know He loves me. And He loves David. Through it all, we trust Him.* She peered once more at the flickering candlelight, and as she slowly squeezed her eyes she watched it spray like warm, colored surf into a thousand particles of dancing color. Light was ahead. *Life* was ahead!

10

Afterward

David stood alone in the cemetery. Moments before Erik and Boris had chased each other on the grass beyond their mother's freshly dug grave, then stood quietly as Scripture was read. The pastor and David's relatives had just driven away. The night before, nearly a thousand people had attended Elsbeth's funeral service.

The March sky was bright and springlike, but a cold wind buffeted David's overcoat. Before him, Lois's white marble stone was separated from Elsbeth's casket only by his great-grandparents' family grave.

Elsbeth had never given up, had never stopped fighting. She had never even given up her passionate sexuality, but with glances and words had communicated her forceful love. She showed such depth of spirit that he felt only Christ could have enriched her personality so greatly. Had not Elsbeth been a gift—a living, joyous gift of color, depth, joy? Were not the years of their love something grief could not crowd out?

"We must pray for a miracle," Elsbeth had declared emphatically the Saturday before she died. How he had longed for one. But he had responded, "What is more of a miracle, to heal your body, or to accept what He is allowing? Which is harder?" And he now knew God had done *that* miracle as she had courageously endured . . . .

The events of the last few days swirled in his mind like the oak leaves—lively, spinning, fluttering against the gravestones, gusting over the high mound of broken, fresh earth.

"Elsbeth, everywhere I go, people are asking how you are," Dr. Gabuzda had told her. "The whole house staff is very proud of you."

Her cancer was the most virulent and aggressive he had ever seen, but her tenacious fighting spirit had kept her alive far beyond his original hopes. "When a patient is dying," a nurse observed, "we usually feel like avoiding the room. But not Elsbeth's. We *want* to be there. Dying is not a time of opening to new people. But Elsbeth kept reaching out to new friends."

She lay unconscious all Friday night. In the morning David was astounded to hear her ask, "Dave, don't you think we should show some slides of Africa tonight?" That evening he set up the projector. She carefully applied White Shoulders perfume behind her ears and on her wrists as if she were going to a concert, then narrated for the nurses. To David's chagrin, however, the projector bulb soon burned out. A helicopter could be heard outside. "Maybe *he's* bringing a bulb," Elsbeth wisecracked through her infected lips, and her audience laughed.

On Sunday David brought Erik and Karba to see Elsbeth. "I love you," Erik told her, then pointing to the sores on her mouth, said, "I'll pray. Thank You dear Lord, bless Mommy, get the boo-boo to go away . . . in Jesus' Name, Amen." Immediately noticing his father's tears, he asked him, "Are you getting sick?"

"A little."

Elsbeth's eyes went to Karba. Erik, seeing her expression, asked his father, "Is she going to cry?" Elsbeth spoke over Erik's voice, "Karba, you listen to Daddy. Okay? He will be a good daddy, and Daddy will help you. When I go to heaven, one day you will go to heaven too. We will see each other again. We don't know when—maybe soon."

"Monday? Saturday?" Erik asked.

"Maybe Jesus is coming very soon," Elsbeth continued. "Maybe you have to wait a little. But I love you. And when I die, I will see Jesus right away. Don't forget, Karba, you have a job to do, just like Erik and Boris. Okay?"

Karba was sitting very quietly, nodding now and then. "Give Mommy a kiss, Karba," David suggested. Erik looked at Karba as she leaned toward her mother. "Is she going to cry, too? Why? Why is she going to cry?"

Afterward

"See, Mommy's going away very soon," David explained. "Mommy is going to heaven, to be with the Lord Jesus."

"Why?"

"Because she is very sick here. She can't stay here any longer. The Lord Jesus wants to take her to be with Him. So Mommy wants us to be good. She wants you to grow up to be a real good boy. She hopes that you will learn to love the Lord Jesus, too, and that you will go to heaven when you die. Okay?"

"Un hummmm."

"Do you want to give Mommy a kiss?"

Erik kissed her and said, "Bye-bye."

"Bye-bye," Elsbeth responded.

Seeing her face, Erik demanded again, "Why is she going to cry?"

"Because we're sad. Our hearts are hurting. When we're sad, we cry. Right?"

"I'm not crying."

"I know. But some day you will." They repeated their good-bye, and Erik added, "I hope you get well. I hope you go down on heaven."

"I'm going to heaven," Elsbeth assured him.

"Good-bye, Mom."

Another day Boris visited her and wrote all over her arm with a red felt-tipped pen. Later someone asked, "What's wrong with your arm, Elsbeth?" "Nothing," she replied. "Those are Boris's marks. That's how he said good-bye."

David knew Elsbeth felt anger and frustration. She felt fear.

God! God! God! she prayed one day, in a near scream. Then, "Jesus Christ! Help me! Help me! Help me believe You understand! Forgive me all my sins."

"Elsbeth, are you sure you're saved?" David questioned.

"Yes, I know," she replied. Then she tilted her head in her unique, little-girl way. "But I am a little afraid."

He read the Scriptures to her that would be read at her funeral. "Do you have peace?" he asked.

She smiled. "Yes. Are you trying to keep me alive?"

"No. We've even stopped the antibiotics."

She smiled again. "I want to die today," she said softly. Then David sang "Precious Lord" to her. "Did you like that?"

"Not really," she admitted, her old feisty spirit showing through again.

She went unconscious. After many hours, as David kept his death-watch, she drifted back to reality and asked, "Dave, why am I still here?"

David moved close to her face. "I don't know, sweetheart. But we can't kill you."

She closed her eyes. "I know."

He sat by her bed. He dozed. Elsbeth was barely breathing. On and on the night went. Suddenly at three o'clock he was startled by Elsbeth's hearty, unrestrained laughter. It awoke him instantly. He jumped up in the dimly lighted room and stared at her. He sensed she was gone, that her eyes were fixed, unseeing; her breathing was a bare movement of the chest, as if her brain and person were gone and the heart was futilely pumping. Had she laughed aloud? He felt enveloped in a rich, wonderful peace, and the echoes of Elsbeth's laughter still reverberated not only in his ears but, somehow, in his entire body.

Had he really heard Elsbeth laugh as she escaped pain and grief—as she saw Jesus and the triumph of heaven? David didn't know or care. Somehow God had given him her laughter, and this enormous peace within was as real as his shirt and jacket.

She stopped breathing at 5:28 A.M. David went out to a nurse and said, "Elsbeth just went home to be with Jesus."

Dr. Kucer, whom Elsbeth had always teased about looking like Dr. Zhivago, entered the room and pronounced her dead. Then he turned to David. "I don't know how to say this, but I just walked into the room and felt such a peace. Why? Usually I'm uncomfortable when I have to pronounce someone dead. But I felt drawn in. I've never seen such peace. Why?"

David, who still felt the peace like a living force inside him, started telling the doctor about how Jesus was her Peace and his, and they talked about Him for a full hour . . . .

Afterward

Workers in nondescript clothes were lowering the casket. David walked away from the gravesite to his car. Keys. Gearshift. Steering wheel. Back to the mundane. He would never completely solve the riddle. Why were their prayers for healing unanswered? As Elsbeth had read their wedding psalm—Psalm 91—she had been increasingly perplexed at the promise of "a thousand may fall at your side, but it shall not come near you." People had "answers" to everything—but they always shimmered above deeper enigmas and mysteries. The only complete reality was the Person of Christ—His Presence and His tasting their pain with them was actual and alive.

He looked at the empty seat beside him and thought of the times they'd sung together while driving. She'd wanted to take voice lessons but now never would. He choked up. He would have to live with such reminders of her. But had not Paul gotten as answer to his own thorn, "My grace is sufficient for thee"? *I trust You, Lord,* he prayed. *You've proven worthy of my trust again and again. You are the all wise, good Creator. Help me realize that You who made the voice probably hear her singing right now. She is alive! More alive than I am!*

He remembered reading the last pages of the book manuscript to her as she lay dying. "She peered once more at the flickering candlelight," he had read, "and as she slowly squeezed her eyes she watched it spray like warm, colored surf into a thousand particles of dancing color. Light was ahead. *Life* was ahead!"

"Is that the way you want the book to end?" he had asked.

"Yes." She had breathed with great difficulty. "I just see it now. When I walked down the aisle, I didn't know where you and Karba sat. Do I walk in my funeral all alone without David and Karba? Do they sit somewhere in the congregation? Here are all the people in front of the casket, mourning. They don't see me walking down to the light, the door to heaven. If they could only see how beautiful it is!"

"If they could only see how beautiful it is."